PHARMACOLOGY - RESEARCH, SAFETY TESTING AND REGULATION

WARFARIN MONITORING

STANDARD PRACTICE AND BEYOND

PHARMACOLOGY - RESEARCH, SAFETY TESTING AND REGULATION

Additional books in this series can be found on Nova's website under the Series tab.

Additional e-books in this series can be found on Nova's website under the e-books tab.

PHARMACOLOGY - RESEARCH, SAFETY TESTING AND REGULATION

WARFARIN MONITORING

STANDARD PRACTICE AND BEYOND

GARY W. MOORE
GRAEME A. THOMSON
AND
DOMINIC J. HARRINGTON

Nova Science Publishers, Inc.
New York

For permission to use material from this book please contact us:
Telephone 631-231-7269; Fax 631-231-8175
Web Site: http://www.novapublishers.com

Library of Congress Cataloging-in-Publication Data

Warfarin monitoring : standard practice and beyond / editors, Gary W. Moore, Graeme Thomson, Dominic J. Harrington.
p. ; cm.
Includes bibliographical references and index.
ISBN 978-1-62100-189-8 (softcover)
I. Moore, Gary, Dr. II. Thomson, Graeme, 1959- III. Harrington, Dominic J.
[DNLM: 1. Warfarin. 2. Drug Monitoring. QV 193]
LC classification not assigned
615.1'9--dc23

2011032450

Published by Nova Science Publishers, Inc. † New York

CONTENTS

PREFACE

Warfarin is one of the most commonly used anticoagulant drugs worldwide with a role in the treatment for a variety of conditions, such as atrial fibrillation, artificial heart valves, deep venous thrombosis, pulmonary embolism and antiphospholipid syndrome. It exerts its anticoagulant effect by interference of the vitamin K mediated γ-carboxylation of the coagulation factors II, VII, IX and X, rendering them dysfunctional by compromising their phospholipid-binding properties. Although effective as an anticoagulant drug, care must be taken in warfarin administration as it interacts with many commonly used medications and some foodstuffs. Additionally, it has a narrow therapeutic range so frequent monitoring with blood tests coupled with expert dose management are crucial to patient safety.

Laboratory monitoring is achieved almost exclusively by use of the prothrombin time (PT). The raw data is converted to the International Normalised Ratio (INR), calculated by division of the patient's clotting time by the local analytical system geometric mean normal PT to generate a PT ratio. This ratio is then taken to the power of a mathematical expression of the sensitivity of the thromboplastin reagent to the warfarin effect relative to an international standard, the International Sensitivity Index (ISI). Theoretically, the INR system should compensate for the inevitable differences in raw clotting times between the vast array of available reagents and analytical platforms. In practice, this can only be the case if laboratories and reagent/analyser manufacturers pay close attention to the variables inherent in INR/ISI assignment. Crucial to accurate INR results is effective local system calibration for each batch of thromboplastin.

The increase in patients requiring anticoagulation has lead to different models of patient management. Traditional hospital-based clinics persist although dosing may be done by suitably trained nurses, pharmacists or scientists as well as medical staff. General practitioners and local pharmacists are increasingly being used in ambulatory based clinics for stable, uncomplicated patients. The advent of point-of-care testing devices for PT/INR determination now allows selected patients to self-test and even self-dose.

Even with effective INR analysis and expert dosing, warfarin is associated with some adverse effects, such as haemorrhage, osteoporosis and purple toe syndrome. Patients with apparent warfarin resistance should be evaluated for compliance, dietary habits and influence of polypharmacy. Genuine warfarin resistance can occur from increased metabolic clearance, decreased absorption or abnormal pharmacodynamics. Heritable warfarin resistance has been described associated with genes coding for components of the cytochrome P450 enzyme system and vitamin K epoxide reductase subunit 1.

When used appropriately and monitored in an informed manner, warfarin can be a cost-effective anticoagulant drug and provide positive patient satisfaction and clinical outcomes.

Chapter 1

DISCOVERY AND MODE OF ACTION OF WARFARIN

INTRODUCTION

Warfarin (Coumadin, Jantoven, Marevan, and Waran), is one of several oral vitamin K antagonists which is clinically used in many conditions including atrial fibrillation, artificial heart valves, deep venous thrombosis, pulmonary embolism, antiphospholipid syndrome and, occasionally, after myocardial infarction. At this time there is great interest in the development of a new generation of oral anticoagulants predominantly based on the direct inhibition of thrombin or activated factor X. In this age of 'modern' drug development it is worth reviewing the discovery of the 4-hydroxycoumarins, of which warfarin is one, a story that unfolded on the prairies of North Dakota and in Alberta, Canada.

DISCOVERY OF AN ORAL ANTICOAGULANT

During the 1920s a fatal haemorrhagic disease afflicting cattle and sheep in North America appeared. The veterinarian Frank Schofield began to study this disease in 1923. He disagreed with the consensus view that the disease was infectious 'black leg' - a usually fatal bacterial disease of cattle and sometimes of sheep, goats, and swine, caused by *Clostridium chauvoe* and characterised by gas-containing swellings in the musculature.

Schofield and a second veterinarian, Lee Roderick, determined that the cause of this disease was not a pathogenic organism or a consequence of a nutritional deficiency but was caused by the feeding of spoilt sweet clover (a consequence of the recent introduction of immigrant farming practices) [1,2]. Cattle and sheep started to exhibit deranged coagulation 15 days after eating the spoiled feed, which would progress to fatal internal haemorrhage between 30 – 50 days later. The bleeding could be prevented by withdrawal of the spoiled sweet clover or by transfusion of fresh blood from healthy animals. By 1931 Roderick showed that the bleeding disorder was a consequence of prothrombin deficiency [3].

Working independently from the veterinarians, in December 1932, Ross Gortner, head of the Biochemistry Department at the University of Minnesota offered a research position to Karl Link. Karl Link had received his PhD in 1925 from the University of Wisconsin working with William Tottingham. He then worked for 2 years in Europe with Sir James Irvine in Scotland; Fritz Pregl in Austria and Paul Karrer in Switzerland – before returning to Wisconsin. One of the projects offered by Prof. Gortner was the study of ‘sweet clover disease’. Link’s initial remit in January 1933 was to work with Professor R.A Brink and Professor W. K Smith in the development of a strain of sweet clover suitable for the climate of Wisconsin that had a low coumarin content. It was known that the bitter taste of green sweet clover (*Melilotus alba* and *Melilotus officianalis*) was correlated with the coumarin content and that cattle had a preference for eating the less bitter plants [4].

One month later the direction of the ‘sweet clover disease’ project was to change as a consequence of a chance encounter on a Saturday afternoon in February 1933. During a blizzard, a farmer called Ed Carlson drove the 190 miles from Deer Park to Wisconsin desperately seeking assistance. The farmer had lost many of his cattle to sweet clover disease after years of using sweet clover without incident. In recent days he had lost several cattle and his bull had begun oozing blood from the nose. He was referred to the Agricultural Experimental Station authorities to learn more but when he arrived at the office with a dead heifer, a milk can containing blood that failed to clot and 100 pounds of feed, it was closed. By chance he met Karl Link. Karl Link was unable to help the farmer and could only reiterate the advice of Roderick and Schofield – stop using the feed and possibly transfuse the cattle that he wanted to save. This chance encounter had an immense impact on Link, the farmer’s dying cattle were a significant loss during the financial depression [5].

Karl Link and his team worked towards isolating, crystallizing and synthesizing the agent in the foodstuff that was causing the deranged coagulation. On the morning of June 28th 1939, Harold Campbell a student from Link's team managed to achieve the crystallisation in the laboratory, referred to as H.A (Haemorrhagic Agent). Mark Stahmann, also a student in the team subsequently managed large scale production, enough for the structure to be elucidated as 3,3'-methylenebis (4-hydroxycoumarin) by Charles Huebner on April 1st 1940 (Figure 1a).

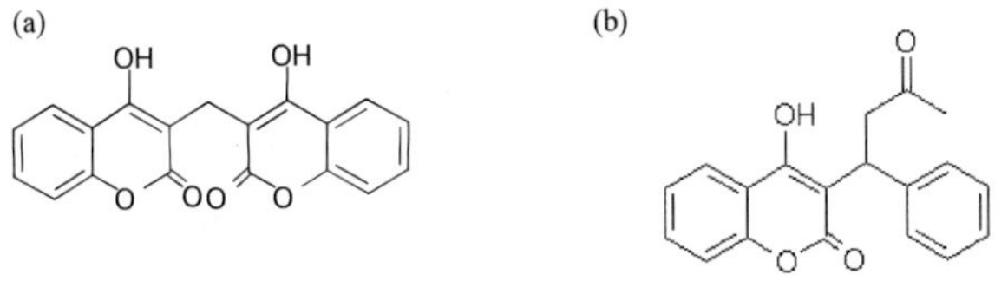

Figure 1. (a) Dicumarol [3,3′-Methyl-bis-(4-hydroxycoumarin)] (b) Warfarin [3- (α-acetonyl-benzyl)-4-hydroxycoumarin].

The spoiling of the sweet clover hay by bacterial action during storage in damp conditions had led to the oxidising of coumarin to 4-hydroxycoumarin which coupled with formaldehyde formed dicumarol. Link gave a lecture about dicumarol to the Mayo clinic on March 12th 1941, and it was there that the substance was first used in an attempt to control thrombotic disorders in humans [6]. Dicumarol was not universally accepted for clinical use immediately. There was controversy over whether vitamin K was an effective antidote, leading to dicumarol being labelled as a dangerous drug. Eventually the tide of evidence changed and it was accepted that vitamin K could reverse the anticoagulant effect. This confusion arose because the prothrombin assays available at the time lacked sufficient sensitivity. A further 10 years were to pass before dicumarol was to lose its reputation in clinical practice as a dangerous drug to be avoided. Link's team went on to synthesise over 150, 4-hydroxycoumarin type compounds some of which were much more potent than dicumarol and at this point the shift in focus was the development of a rodenticide. Trials found that dicumarol failed to induce a state of vitamin K deficiency in rats to a degree sufficient to control populations. Link's team compared the various 4-hydroxycoumarin analogues using the following criteria [5]:

- degree of purity that could be easily achieved
- absence of taste and odour
- production costs
- whether they could be converted to a stable water-soluble salt

After reviewing the comparative data in 1948 (during a period of ill health and a prolonged period of recuperation), Link proposed compound no. 42 for rodenticide use (3-(α-acetonyl-benzyl)-4-hydroxycoumarin (Figure 1b). This view was contrary to the consensus of his laboratory team who favoured a direct derivative of no 42 – analogue no. 63. Analogue no. 42 was marketed by the Wisconsin research foundation by Ward Ross (General Manager). Link coined the name using the first letters of **W**isconsin **A**lumni **R**esearch **F**oundation with *arin* to reflect its coumarin origins. In late 1950, Link suggested to Dr Shepard Shapiro (a pioneer of therapeutic dicumarol use) and Dr Ovid Meyer (who had reviewed analogue no. 63) that warfarin would be well suited to clinical use. Making the transition from rodenticide to clinical use proved difficult and the medical community were reluctant to use warfarin. On April 5th 1951 Link and his team were informed that an army recruit had been admitted to the Naval Hospital having taken a large dose of warfarin intended for rodenticide use. The patient had been given a blood transfusion and vitamin K and then made a full recovery [4]. This incident acted as a catalyst for studies into the use of warfarin as a therapeutic agent and in 1954 warfarin was approved for medical use in humans. An early recipient was US president Dwight Eisenhower, who was prescribed warfarin after experiencing a heart attack in 1955 [4]. More than half a century later, warfarin remains the most widely prescribed oral anticoagulant [7].

Mode of Action

The mechanism behind the action of warfarin was not elucidated until Bell and Matschiner reported that warfarin increased the amount of circulatory vitamin K_1 2,3-epoxide (K_1O) relative to vitamin K_1 (K_1) [8], whose structural formulae are shown in Figure 2. Later, after the discovery of vitamin K epoxide reductase, it was found that this enzyme was inhibited by warfarin [9].

Warfarin exerts its anticoagulant effect by preventing the conversion of specific glutamate residues within the vitamin K-dependent coagulation factors (II, VII, IX, X) to γ-carboxyglutamate (Gla). Located within the first 40 residues of each mature protein (known as the Gla domain) are 9 – 13 Gla residues, of which the first 9 are fully conserved and the 10th is highly conserved. Gla is a metal binding amino acid that confers metal binding properties on vitamin K-dependent proteins. The binding of calcium ions induces two sequential conformational changes that expose a phospholipid binding site, which in association with an adjacent aromatic amino acid stack domain enables attachment of these proteins to phospolipid membranes during coagulation factor activation [10] (Figure 3.).

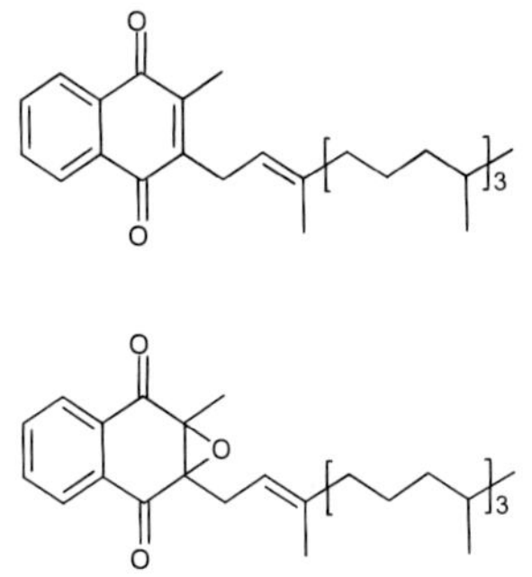

Phylloquinone (vitamin K_1)

Vitamin K_1 2,3-epoxide

Figure 2. Structural formulae of vitamin K_1 and vitamin K_1 2,3-epoxide.

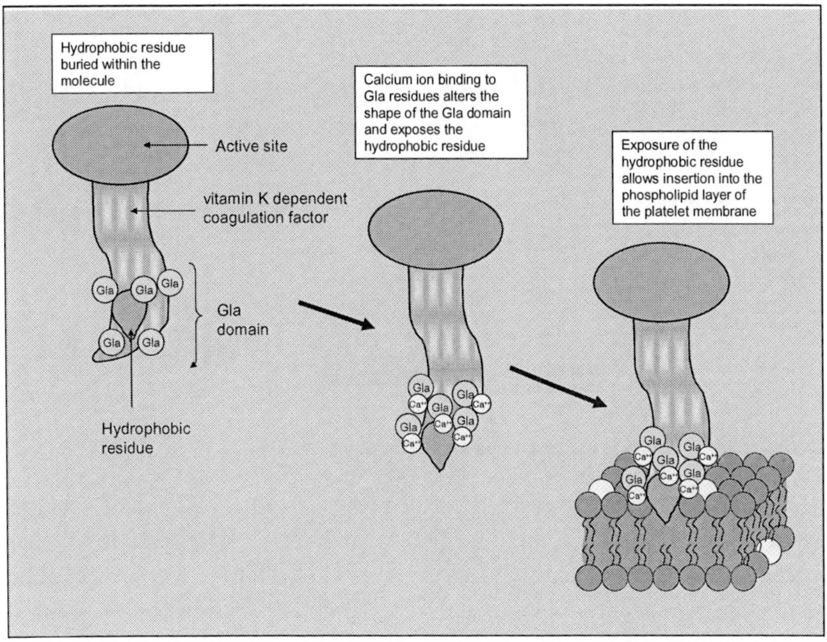

Figure 3. Gla domain function in vitamin K dependent coagulation factors. Gla domains are internalised upon binding of Ca^{++} and hydrophobic residues that were masked by the Gla domains become exposed, permitting penetration of the phospholipid membrane and further interactions between protein and negatively charged phospholipid. Reproduced with permission from Oxford University Press, UK [11].

Several divalent metal ions induce the first conformational change but the second is only supported by calcium ions.

The genes that encode these proteins share significant organisational similarity and evolved from a common ancestral gene [12]. This conversion is performed by the liver microsomal enzyme γ-glutamyl carboxylase that requires the reduced form of vitamin K (vitamin K hydroquinone; abbreviated (KH_2)) as a co-factor.

During the γ-carboxylation reaction, KH_2 is converted to its epoxide form. A second enzyme termed the vitamin K epoxide reductase complex (VKORC) recycles vitamin K epoxide back to KH_2, helping to provide sufficient cofactor for subsequent γ-carboxylation reactions (Figure 4.).

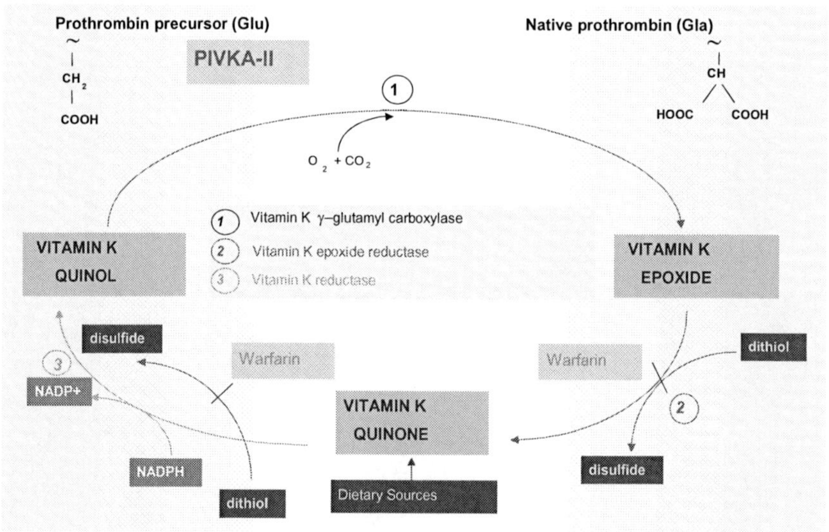

Figure 4. The vitamin K cycle and associated enzymes.

Warfarin inhibits the VKORC and prevents the salvaging of vitamin K epoxide. This leads to a rapid depletion of hepatic KH_2 availability and a decrease in γ-glutamyl carboxylase activity [13]. During warfarin treatment, vitamin K-dependent factors with incompletely carboxylated glutamate residues, known as **P**roteins **I**nduced by **V**itamin **K** **A**bsence or antagonism (**PIVKA**) are released into the circulation. Fully carboxylated glutamate residues are required for full functionality of the vitamin K dependent clotting factors and the corresponding PIVKAs show greatly reduced coagulation activity.

Chapter 2

STANDARD LABORATORY MONITORING OF WARFARIN

PROTHROMBIN TIME

The most commonly used laboratory test for monitoring of warfarin is the prothrombin time (PT) that was first described by Quick in 1935 [14,15]. This was before the discovery of oral anticoagulants and it was initially introduced as a screening test for coagulation defects, for which it is still used. The PT has undergone a variety of modifications since its original description yet the basic principle remains.

PRINCIPLE AND PERFORMANCE OF THE PROTHROMBIN TIME

Although the cascade theory of coagulation biochemistry has been superseded by the cell surface-based model for *in vivo* coagulation [16], the PT and its screening test counterpart the activated partial thromboplastin time (APTT) are designed with the cascade theory as their backdrop. The nature of the reagents used to initiate *in vitro* coagulation are such that the PT initiates coagulation exclusively via the 'extrinsic' pathway whereas the APTT does so via the 'intrinsic' pathway. Both pathways generate activated factor X (FXa) which begins the 'common' pathway, thereby generating a fibrin clot as the measurable end point. A basic outline of the coagulation cascade is shown in Figure 5 depicting the separate compartments.

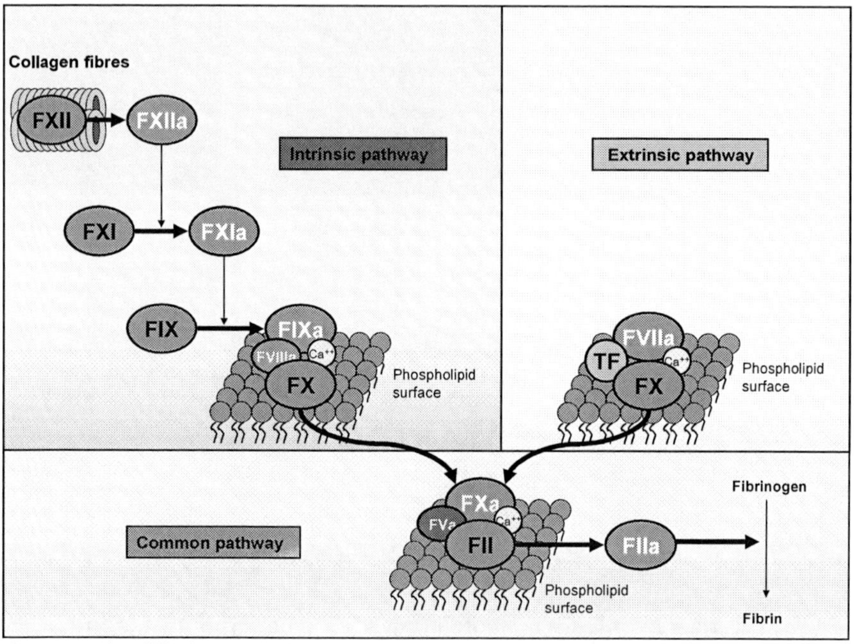

Figure 5. Simplified coagulation cascade theory. The intrinsic pathway is activated by contact of the zymogen factor XII with negatively charged collagen, converting it to the active enzyme FXIIa which activates the next zymogen in the pathway, FXI. A cascade of activation of subsequent zymogens ensues culminating in generation of thrombin (FIIa) which acts on fibrinogen to generate the fibrin clot. The extrinsic pathway merely consists of activation of factor VII to generate activated FX which then enters the common pathway. Note that the activated vitamin K dependent factors VII, IX and X require the presence of a phospholipid surface and calcium ions, and the co-factors of tissue factor, FVIIIa and FVa respectively. Reproduced with permission from Oxford University Press, UK [17].

The PT measures the time a patient's plasma takes to clot in the presence of optimal concentrations of tissue factor, phospholipid and calcium ions. No activator of the intrinsic pathway is contained in the assay system so factor XII remains dormant and subsequent components of that pathway are not activated. The tissue factor facilitates activation of factor VII thereby allowing formation of the extrinsic tenase complex, which consists of the active enzyme FVIIa and its co-factor and substrate, tissue factor and factor X respectively, in the presence of calcium ions on a phospholipid surface. The product of this reaction is FXa, which is the active enzyme of the prothrombinase complex, which also contains FVa as the cofactor for FXa and factor II (prothrombin) as its substrate. This also occurs in the presence of calcium ions on a phospholipid surface. The product of this reaction is FIIa (thrombin) which cleaves small peptides from fibrinogen to expose acceptor sites which then join with donor sites on adjacent molecules to form insoluble fibrin polymers – the fibrin clot.

The clotting time obtained when performing a PT thus reflects the combined activities of three vitamin K dependent factors (factors II, VII and X) and two non-vitamin K dependent factors, factor V and fibrinogen. However, reductions in fibrinogen activity need to be marked before they will prolong a PT (<1.0g/L) and factor V deficiency is extremely rare, so the major determinants of the clotting times are vitamin K dependent factors, making PT a potentially ideal tool for warfarin monitoring.

The significance of the calcium ions and phospholipid is that they are crucial to *in vivo* localisation mechanisms via the interactions with Gla domains described earlier. Thus, fibrin is formed only where it is needed in order to strengthen platelet clots that would otherwise be haemostatically ineffective in parts of the circulatory system that experience high sheer stress.

Crucial to performance of a PT is the thromboplastin reagent, the source of both the tissue factor and phospholipid in the reaction mixture [18]. The original thromboplastin used by Quick was prepared from rabbit brain, the brain of course being an organ rich in both tissue factor and lipids. Other tissues have since been used as a source of thromboplastin, such as human, bovine or rabbit brain, rabbit lung and human placenta. Human brain thromboplastins were the most widely used initially as they could be prepared locally by each laboratory using readily available cadaver brains from the hospital mortuary. However, there was no inter-institution standardisation for thromboplastin preparation and use, and unsurprisingly, there was significant variation of laboratory results. The 1950s saw the introduction of commercial supplies of thromboplastin which relieved hospital staff of the burden of regular reagent preparation and a greater degree of standardisation was assumed. Not having such a wide access to human brains, commercial manufacturers took to preparing thromboplastins from the other sources as well as human brain.

The early 1960s brought recognition that despite the availability of commercial thromboplastins there was poor inter-laboratory agreement in PT results. This was partly explained by use of reagents prepared from different species, further complicated by contamination with serum containing factors II, VII and X – the very vitamin K dependent factors the PT assesses when used for warfarin monitoring. This made the reagents less responsive to the effects of warfarin and lead to unwarranted increases in dose to achieve target PT values and a subsequent increase in bleeding episodes. Thromboplastins from the same tissue source also exhibited considerable differences. Clearly, improvements in inter-batch thromboplastin standardisation and inter-laboratory agreement, both nationally and internationally, were necessary to achieve more robust and effective warfarin management and improvement in patient care. A patient should get a sufficiently similar result wherever their analysis is performed so that clinicians can dose accordingly.

The first attempt at PT standardisation was made in Manchester in the UK in 1962 when a standardised thromboplastin comprising phenolised human brain extract was supplied to laboratories in that area [19]. By 1969, the technique for large scale production of thromboplastin with nearly identical performance between successive batches meant that the Manchester Comparative Reagent (MCR) was adopted as the national reagent. A common reporting system was adopted, the British Ratio, whereby the patient PT with MCR was divided by that of the PT of a normal pooled control plasma with MCR. For hospitals not using MCR, batches of MCR were designated as reference preparations and re-named British Comparative Reagent for comparison with locally prepared or alternative commercial reagents. Virtually every hospital in the UK was using MCR by the mid-1970s but it was not possible to supply such a reagent to other countries, so alternative models were needed to standardise PT testing/warfarin dosing worldwide.

An identical reagent could not be supplied to every laboratory worldwide so a system was needed to calibrate thromboplastins from different tissues and species. A number of models were considered, such as the Biggs-Denson calibration model of equivalent ratios, but were not adopted. An international collaborative study was published by the International Committee on Thrombosis and Haemostasis in 1979 which lead to the proposal of the International Normalised Ratio (INR) system, which was adopted as the World Health Organisation (WHO) international PT standardisation scheme in 1983.

Native human brain preparations were withdrawn from general use in 1986, mainly due to potential risks of infection during manufacture, in particular, Creutzfeldt-Jakob disease and human immunodeficiency virus. They were initially replaced by rabbit brain thromboplastins that caused concern about comparability with human brain-derived reagents, mainly as a result of reduced sensitivity to the warfarin effect. Sensitive rabbit brain thromboplastins are now available. The early 1990s saw the availability of thromboplastin reagents containing highly purified recombinant human tissue factor produced in *E. Coli* reconstituted into synthetic phospholipid vesicles. To function effectively in coagulation the vesicles contain phospholipids with a net negative charge, the most effective being phosphatidyl serine.

Consequently, recombinant thromboplastins are composed entirely of defined ingredients and are thus potentially superior to the relatively crude tissue extract reagents of human or animal origin.

The International Normalised Ratio

The INR is based on a mathematical relationship between the PT ratio of a patient's plasma analysed using a given thromboplastin with the PT ratio that would have been obtained with the original WHO standard thromboplastin. The PT ratio is calculated from dividing the PT by a previously determined geometric mean normal prothrombin time (GMNPT) for that thromboplastin. The relationship between the thromboplastin in local use and the WHO standard is defined by a numerical value, the International Sensitivity Index (ISI). The INR is calculated as follows:

$$\left[\frac{\text{Patient PT (s)}}{\text{GMNPT (s)}}\right]$$

Crucial to generation of accurate INRs, that is to say, the PT ratio that would be obtained if the WHO standard thromboplastin was used, is accurate ISI assignment. The ISI is a measure of the responsiveness of a thromboplastin to the oral anticoagulant effect relative to the WHO standard. ISIs are assigned to thromboplastins after calibration against the WHO standard or a secondary standard that has been calibrated against it.

Thromboplastin Calibration and ISI Assignment

The original so-called international reference preparation (IRP), designated 67/40, was a human brain extract and is no longer available. All subsequent IRPs have had their ISIs defined in terms of 67/40 although there is an inevitable degree of uncertainty in the accuracy of ISI assignment. This is limited by assigning ISIs to new IRPs using large, multicentre calibration exercises involving collaboration between 20 laboratories or more from different countries (>10). Currently, WHO standard preparations exist for thromboplastins of recombinant human, native rabbit or native bovine origin.

The bovine standard is the only one that was directly compared to 67/40. Interestingly, 67/40 was a 'combined' reagent, so-called because adsorbed bovine plasma had been added to optimise factor V and fibrinogen content. Adsorption with aluminium hydroxide removes vitamin K dependent factors thus making such thromboplastins ideal for oral anticoagulant monitoring but unusable for diagnostic use. All subsequent human and rabbit IRPs have been plain thromboplastins (no addition of adsorbed plasma) and bovine IRPs combined thromboplastins. Commercial thromboplastins tend to double as diagnostic reagents and are usually plain reagents unless specifically marketed for oral anticoagulant monitoring.

Irrespective of type, any new IRP is calibrated against all existing IRPs. The ISI assigned to the new IRP is taken as the mean ISI obtained from the calibration with each current IRP. A typical procedure would be as follows; each collaborating centre identifies 20 healthy individuals and 60 patients stabilised on oral anticoagulation for at least 6 weeks with INRs in the range 1.5 – 4.5. These are considered the minimum numbers required for an accurate calibration. Over a 10 day period, fresh plasma samples from two of the healthy individuals and six of the orally anticoagulated patients are tested by prothrombin time with each of the existing IRPs and the IRP being calibrated. PTs on each sample are typically performed in quadruplicate. An orthogonal regression line is prepared on the basis of the natural logarithms of the PTs. The results for the IRP are plotted on the vertical axis and those for the preparation being calibrated on the horizontal axis as shown in Figure 6. The model provides an estimate of the standard deviation of data points about the regression line, thus it is important to remove the results from any sample with a perpendicular distance greater than three residual standard deviations from the regression line.

The orthogonal regression model assumes that a single line describes the relationship between log(PT) of both populations yet you can see in Figure 6 that there may be deviation between a calibration line drawn through the normal + abnormal populations and one drawn through the abnormals only. Lack of coincidence can be corrected using Tomenson's correction calculation [20]. For practical purposes where deviation remains marked, an ISI can still be assigned if INRs calculated with the ISI derived from the overall regression line are within 10% of INRs calculated from the regression line for the abnormals only, in the INR range 2.0 – 4.5.

The slope of the orthogonal regression line through both populations is used to calculate the ISI of the new IRP.

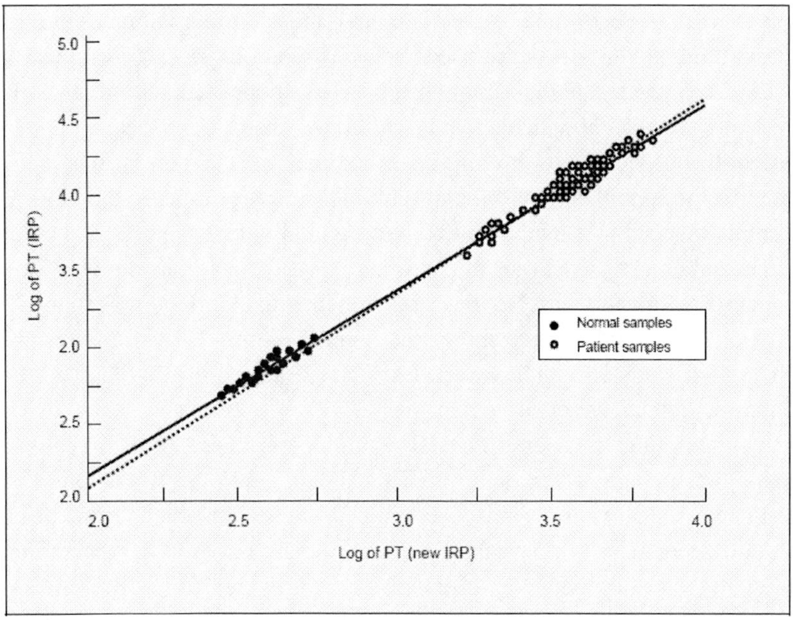

Figure 6. Plot of log of prothrombin times for ISI determination. Continuous line represents structural relation for normal and orally anticoagulated patient samples and dotted line for patients only.

The reader is referred to the WHO technical report '*Guidelines for thromboplastins and plasma used to control oral anticoagulant therapy*' for details of the calculations used to derive the ISI from the slope of the orthogonal regression line. (http://www.who.int/bloodproducts/ publications/ WHO_TRS_889_A3.pdf)

Secondary standards, such as national reference preparations and manufacturer's working standards, should be calibrated against the IRP for the corresponding species. It is not practical to undertake large, multicentre calibration exercises for secondary standards but WHO recommends that the exercise is performed by at least two laboratories to minimise the effects of interlaboratory variation. These secondary standards are used to calibrate manufacturers' commercial reagents. Each new batch of reagent should be calibrated against a thromboplastin from the same tissue of the same species that has been prepared using a similar manufacturing process. The calibration is usually undertaken using pooled normal plasmas and pooled plasmas from orally anticoagulated patients. Plasmas artificially depleted of vitamin K dependent factors are also available. Use of pooled plasmas means that the numbers of PTs performed to generate the regression line is much less than if fresh individual samples were used. Some workers have advocated use of as few as three plasma pools although this would depend on the quality of the pools and the thromboplastin being calibrated. Data point scatter about the regression line tends to be minimal because of the similarities between calibrator thromboplastin and the thromboplastin reagent being calibrated, and also reduction of biological variation between individual samples by pooling.

Thromboplastins with an ISI between 0.9 – 1.7 are considered to possess acceptable responsiveness to the oral anticoagulant effect for clinical use. However, some studies have shown that interlaboratory ISI variation is greater with high ISI systems than low ISI systems, suggesting that INRs are less accurate with the less sensitive reagents.

It is tempting to assume that all manufacturers need to do is calibrate a thromboplastin against an appropriate standard and supply customers with batch-specific ISI values. This does indeed happen in practice but does not take into account all the variables that can impact on PT/INR generation. As well as the variation between thromboplastins prepared from different species and tissues, another important variable that impacts on clotting times is the analytical method used to deliver reagents and detect the fibrin clot end point. There are three methods in common use for end point detection that can also vary in their reagent delivery options:

Tilt-tube technique: Reagents and plasma are manually pipetted into test tubes in a 37°C water bath and the time taken to clot estimated using a stopwatch. The test tube is removed from the water bath, held horizontally and returned 2-3 times/second until the reaction mixture is seen to have clotted. The advent of automated analytical systems has caused a marked decline in use of this technique. It remains the reference method but is inappropriate to the high workloads of many hospital laboratories.

Mechanical clot detection: Reagents and plasma are manually pipetted into rotating, angled cuvettes containing a metal ball sitting within a magnetic field. The cuvettes are contained within a coagulometer that reads the end point when formation of the fibrin clot removes the metal ball from the magnetic field. Automated versions are available that use robotics to deliver reagents and plasma and time to clot formation.

Photo-optical clot detection: Reagents and plasma are delivered by robotics and end-points are timed automatically. Reaction cuvettes are placed in a light path and the increase in turbidity upon fibrin formation alters the light-scatter which is detected photo-optically by either nephelometry or turbidimetry.

Each of the methods has innate limitations that impact on the clotting time, even if the same plasma sample and thromboplastin are used for analysis by each method. The tilt-tube technique in particular is prone to operator variability as is the semi-manual version of the mechanical technique, albeit to a lesser extent. Robotic reagent and plasma delivery with automated clot detection has much less variability although that property is reliant on regular and effective equipment maintenance. Accuracy of photo-optical clot detection can be compromised if the plasma has properties that will alter light scatter, such as haemolysis, icterus or lipaemia. The increased plasma viscosity of a markedly lipaemic sample can compromise mechanical clot detection as can formation of a weak clot.

Manual and semi-manual techniques involve incubating plasma with thromboplastin until both have reached reaction temperature before adding calcium ions and beginning timing for clot formation. This negates the need to keep a thromboplastin reagent at 37°C which would otherwise increase the speed of reagent deterioration. Automated techniques use thromboplastin reagents containing calcium ions because the reagent pool can be maintained in a cooled compartment and the aliquot used for each test heated immediately prior to dispensing into the test plasma. Photo-optical clot detection is more sensitive to fibrin clot end point detection than mechanical clot detection, which in turn is more sensitive than the manual tilt tube technique, so even when discounting other interfering factors, all three methods will generate different clotting times with the same sample and reagent.

Clearly, use of the same ISI for a given thromboplastin on different analytical systems is inappropriate because the variation in raw clotting time for a given sample will generate a different INR by each method. Interestingly, IRPs are calibrated using the tilt-tube technique performed by one expert operator, (that is how 67/40 was tested), yet the vast majority of hospital laboratories employ fully automated PT analyses in order to cope with high workloads. Consequently, it is essential that laboratories undertake their own local system ISI calibration for each new batch of thromboplastin that takes into account the specific reagent/technique/end-point detection method(s) in local use [21,22]. Laboratories with more than one technique/analyser should calibrate the reagent for each one even if they are the same type and model. Some manufacturers do provide instrument-specific ISIs but local-system ISI should still be undertaken to account for local variations in technique and maintenance procedures.

A study by Chantarangkul *et al* demonstrated that a reliable local system ISI can be derived from a minimum of seven normal and 20 abnormal plasmas

[23]. Those numbers of samples are necessary for high ISI reagents but it has been shown that a minimum of three normals and 10 abnormals can be used for low ISI reagents [14]. The European Concerted Action on Anticoagulation (ECAA) provides certified sets of seven normal and 20 artificially depleted lyophilised plasmas for local system ISI calibration that are described as 'substantially equivalent to a full fresh plasma ISI calibration.' However, some would contend this and prefer to use fresh plasmas, mainly because the freeze drying process can prolong prothrombin times in normal and abnormal plasmas when analysed with a low ISI thromboplastin. In practice, obtaining sufficient numbers of fresh plasmas from normal and orally anticoagulated donors on a regular basis is prohibitive for most hospital laboratories so use of so-called certified plasmas obtained from manufacturers or reference centres, such as the ECAA set, is commonplace. Similarly, obtaining sufficient quantities of plasma from orally anticoagulated patients throughout the 2.0–4.5 range of INRs is difficult for manufacturers and use of lyophilised, artificially depleted plasmas continues. Some manufacturers do supply lyophilised pools prepared from plasma of stably orally anticoagulated donors.

The ECAA plasmas, or similar products from other manufacturers, are each assigned a PT value by the manufacturer using a manual technique employing an IRP thromboplastin [24]. The local laboratory performs PTs in quadruplicate on each plasma with their reagent/technique/end-point detection method in the same working session and the ISI determined as described above.

Alternative plasma sets are available for which the certified plasmas are assigned INR values from a manual method using a reference thromboplastin [24]. The PTs are analysed by local procedures and the logs of the PTs are plotted against the logs of the reference INR as shown in Figure 5. The INRs of patient's plasmas can then be generated from local PT analysis by direct interpolation from the orthogonal regression line, thereby negating the need for determination of ISI or GMNPT. Note in Figure 7 that the regression line is generated from a small number of samples because each one is a pool. For this method, PTs should be determined in duplicate with the local procedures and repeated on at least three separate occasions to allow for day-to-day variation.

The effect of lyophilisation has a variable effect on ISI calibration depending on the method of freeze-drying employed and the reagent /technique/analyser combination in local use [25]. The changes to plasma during the freeze-drying process can be reduced if plasma is buffered shortly after collection but not eliminated.

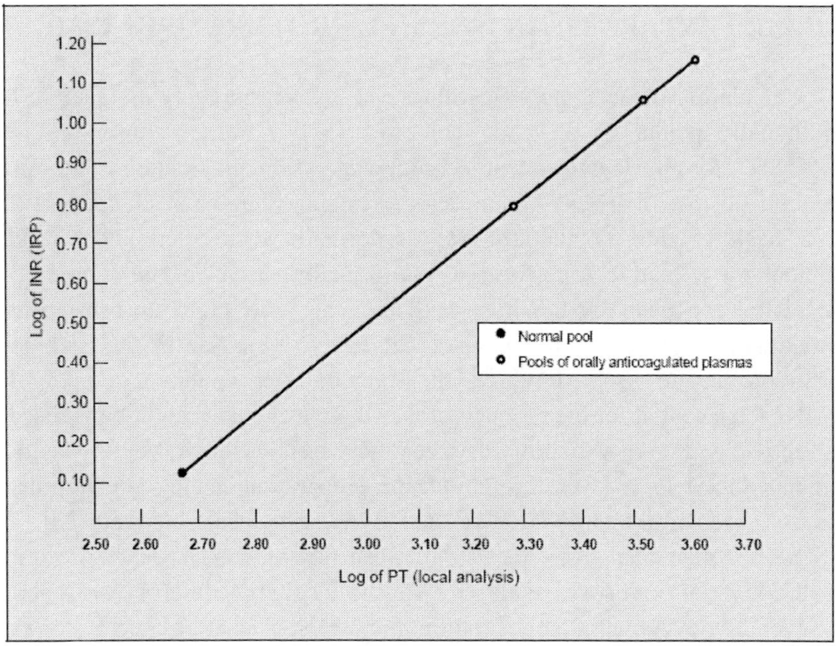

Figure 7. Direct INR measurement calibration line.

Consequently, frozen plasmas are also available for local system ISI calibration as the INR of fresh plasmas is largely unchanged on freezing. Frozen plasmas tend to show a lower degree of INR variability between thromboplastins [26] but there are logistical difficulties in preserving sample integrity during shipment and storage and increased costs when doing so.

Actual PT values of certified plasmas will differ depending on the species of thromboplastin used so each plasma should be certified for the different species. Theoretically, this should not be necessary for the direct INR determination because the INR system itself exists to minimise/eradicate these differences.

In practice, some freeze-dried plasmas have exhibited differences between thromboplastins, and if those discrepancies are marked, that particular certified plasma/thromboplastin combination may be unsuitable. Manufacturers of certified plasmas should specify the reagent/analyser combinations for which their products have been shown to operate reliably. Wherever possible, local ISI should be derived using certified values derived from the same species thromboplastin.

Geometric Mean Normal Prothrombin Time

Calculation of accurate INR values via an appropriately assigned ISI is additionally reliant on a valid geometric mean normal prothrombin time (GMNPT) for the local reagent/technique/analyser combination. The WHO recommends use of GMNPT in preference to an arithmetic mean because PTs in a healthy adult population are log-normally distributed and GMNPT calculations effectively perform a log transformation of the data before calculating the mean itself. Whilst mathematically correct, in most instances it provides little or no significant practical benefit over use of the arithmetic mean or median [27]. However, most laboratories continue to apply the GMNPT to account for the rare occasions where its benefit might be realised.

In recognition of variability between local systems, any GMNPT stated by a manufacturer for a given thromboplastin preparation cannot be extrapolated for local use and the GMNPT, like the ISI, must be locally derived [28]. The GMNPT is generated from the PTs of fresh plasma from at least 20 normal adult donors of both sexes analysed with the local procedure(s) over a period of several days. As with ISI generation, the GMNPT must be specific for each analyser even if the same type and model. Sophisticated analytical equipment deteriorates over time, even when receiving regular and effective maintenance, so GMNPT may alter over time. The changes should however be minimal but re-assessment of GMNPT should not be overlooked if internal or external quality control schemes indicate deterioration in PT/INR performance. Both GMNPT and ISI should be re-assessed following major service of equipment.

Strictly speaking, the GMNPT should be locally assessed for each new batch of thromboplastin but many laboratories do not have the resources or donor availability to do so. One solution to the problem of local donor availability is to calculate the GMNPT from the PT and INR of a lyophilised or frozen pooled normal plasma obtained during the ISI calibration exercise. The normal plasma pool should be prepared from a large number of donors, some currently on the market using in excess of 100. The calculated GMNPT is a theoretical value based on the assumption that the PT of such a large pool should indeed give a PT identical to the GMNPT. The calculation is as follows:

$$\text{Theoretical GMNPT} = \frac{\text{PT of normal pooled plasma (s)}}{\text{INR of normal pooled plasma}}$$

Lyophilised or frozen plasmas can only be substituted for fresh plasmas if the laboratory has shown that the mean result of replicate PTs of lyophilised or frozen plasmas analysed by local procedures is identical to that of fresh plasma samples.

POINT OF CARE TESTING

The majority of clinical laboratories adopt automated equipment for performance of routine coagulation screening tests in order to effectively accommodate high workloads. However, it is not always logistically possible to deliver the fast turnaround of INR results required in many busy anticoagulant clinics from a remote centralised laboratory and point of care testing (POCT) with portable analytical devices is a commonly adopted model to address this issue. This enables laboratory scientists to deliver INR results within the environs of the clinic itself.

POCT devices for INR determination are available from a number of manufacturers that are effectively semi-manual analysers in that reagents and blood samples are loaded manually and end-point detection is automatic. Most of them are designed to perform PT/INR on whole blood samples from capillary punctures although many can also analyse plasma. Thromboplastin reagents are provided in a dry state on disposable test strips or within cartridges that are inserted into the analyser upon addition of the whole blood sample. In view of their specific use in oral anticoagulant monitoring some thromboplastins are of the 'combined' variety. Fresh capillary puncture samples typically contain sufficient calcium ions to facilitate *in vitro* coagulation and some strips/cartridges do not contain calcium reagent, although there are others that do. Separate strips/cartridges are also available for testing citrated venous whole blood or plasma and they inevitably contain calcium ions.

A variety of clot detection principles have been adopted for POCT instruments. The main methods are summarised below:

- Red cell motion slows and stops as whole blood begins to clot and is detected using optical pattern recognition by changes in laser interference.
- Paramagnetic iron oxide particles pulsate within alternating magnetic fields. Their motion slows and stops as blood clots and is detected optically.

- The change in position of a magnet in a slowly rotating reaction tube is detected when clot formation removes it from a magnetic field.
- Whole blood is pumped back and forth inside small bore channels. Reduction in fluid oscillation as blood clots is detected photo-optically.
- The thrombin generated during clot formation reacts with a fluorescent substrate.
- Clot formation is detected by a change in electrical impedance of the blood that occurs when fibrinogen is converted to fibrin.

Numerous studies have been published comparing individual or groups of POCT analysers against each other and more standard laboratory equipment. In view of the variety of clot detection methods available and recognised variable responsiveness of thromboplastin reagents, it is perhaps unsurprising that differences have been reported in INR results [29]. Some studies have concluded that the POCT devices being evaluated demonstrated high concordance with the chosen standard analysis [30,31] whilst others have reported systematic bias [32,33] or agreement only up to INR values between 3.0 – 4.0 [34,35]. An important consideration is that although two methods may be statistically different, the magnitude of difference may be small enough that dosage decisions are not markedly affected and the methods can be considered clinically equivalent. This has been the conclusion of some studies although others have suggested that results beyond the therapeutic range may not be reliable, or at least, may not agree with standard testing. An institution using POCT in outpatient anticoagulant clinics should be aware of the degree of correlation between the POCT device and the standard method(s) employed in the centralised laboratory. Analytical parity within the therapeutic range is important because patients may be tested by both methods during a given period of anticoagulation [29]. Discordance between POCT devices and standard testing tends to be greater with INRs above the therapeutic range and it is common for such POCT results to be checked with a venous sample with standard testing before decisions are made about reversal options.

As well as the recognised differences between thromboplastins and end-point detection systems, POCT devices have additional dimensions that impact on result variability. The thromboplastin in standard reagents that is reacted with plasma is in liquid form so the factor VII only encounters a stable, fully hydrated reagent. The dry reagent in the POCT test strips/cartridges, however, is only reconstituted upon contact with the blood sample itself meaning that the factor VII is exposed to thromboplastin in intermediate states, which can affect the clotting time [36]. This effect can be reduced by use of recombinant thromboplastin reagents as they have a uniform and defined micelle composition and thus a sharp phase transition upon reconstitution. Tissue thromboplastins consist of a heterogeneous population of micelles and hence a poorly defined phase transition. The transition of recombinant thromboplastins from dry to liquid state is therefore more consistent, resulting in factor VII encountering a more uniformly reacting reagent and improved analytical accuracy. The reconstitution of thromboplastin at the start of the reaction can result in longer clotting times than seen in plasma samples receiving standard analysis. In contrast to typical PT testing where end-point detection is the first appearance of measurable clot formation, many POCT instruments take readings beyond this point and determine the time of initial onset by extrapolation or interpolation. POCT devices incorporate internal calculations in order to generate results that better correlate with standard testing.

Local system ISI assignment poses significant logistical difficulties for hospital laboratories as POCT devices require a calibration exercise of similar complexity to that of a secondary standard. The requirement to calibrate using fresh capillary blood on a large number of normal donors and orally anticoagulated patients with a range of INRs makes it a prohibitive exercise. As a result, batches of test strips/cartridges are typically calibrated by the manufacturer against an IRP and the consequent ISI is adopted by all users. To a large extent it is a local system ISI as users will be employing the same reagent and POCT device, although operator and individual device variability are not accounted for. The ECAA has developed simplified ISI calibration procedures for certain POCT instruments yet they involve calibration with lyophilised plasmas and not whole blood.

The portability and relative ease of use of POCT instruments has lead to their operation by non-laboratory personnel such as nurses and pharmacists in clinics and primary care settings. This model has proven acceptable in many institutions providing that adequate initial and refresher training and quality control procedures are in place. Many hospitals have POCT committees to ensure acceptable analytical and clinical quality standards are maintained, and support is usually available from the centralised laboratory. Advice is available from both sources on selection of suitable instruments.

The increase in clinical indications for oral anticoagulant therapy and consequent additional demands on monitoring services has been one of the drivers for introduction of patient self-testing and even management. Furthermore, some patients seek more autonomy and control of their condition as well as issues of convenience. The majority of studies assessing relative clinical safety and efficacy of patient self-management compared to conventional models have concluded that the former is comparable or even superior to the latter in terms of time spent within target INR range, adverse events and outcome [37-39]. Whilst this may be encouraging at first sight, caution must be advised when considering patient self-management as a local option. Not all patients are willing to undertake self monitoring or can be successfully trained to do so, especially for long-term anticoagulation. Equally, short term anticoagulation doesn't necessarily lend itself to patient self management as there is insufficient time to gain familiarity. The quality of training is crucial to effective self management and the formalised training programme in Germany utilising training centres throughout the country has been a particularly successful model.

Cost effectiveness of patient self management has two main dimensions. Providing large numbers of patients with individual POCT devices and associated consumables results in a considerable increase in cost of anticoagulant monitoring, especially bearing in mind that a degree of liaison and follow-up via conventional settings is inevitable. If the findings of studies claiming reduction of thromboembolic or haemorrhagic complications can be widely reproduced then the additional costs associated with provision of home monitoring may be offset or even result in substantial overall cost savings for health providers.

Quality Assurance

Quality assurance of course relates to every activity that contributes to the delivery of reliable test results, from the choice of appropriate tests/reagents/equipment through effective on-going training and education of both users and providers, to effective laboratory practice on a day-to-day basis. Laboratories delivering monitoring services must familiarise themselves with the issues of variability between local systems and the importance of correct assignment of ISI and GMNPT parameters and implement appropriate procedures.

On a day-to-day operational basis, regular maintenance procedures are essential to optimise performance of automated, semi-automated and POCT equipment. Internal quality control (IQC) employing periodical analysis of specially prepared materials throughout the day ensures continual evaluation of reagent, analyser and operator performance. Control material is usually in the form of lyophilised or frozen commercially prepared plasmas which are assigned an expected range of results, which may be specific to particular reagent and/or analyser types. An isolated control result with the local system that is within the range would normally indicate that the local system is functioning adequately. Cumulative control results are statistically evaluated, commonly with a Levy-Jennings plot, to assess for the appearance of trends or bias. Wherever possible, IQC should include control samples with normal and abnormal results to ensure that local analysis detects normality and otherwise.

IQC for POCT instruments presents unique difficulties because a commercial supply of fresh non-anticoagulated whole blood with an assigned result range is patently unfeasible. Consequently, many manufacturers supply liquid control material that can be analysed using test strip/cartidges. This serves to check analyser performance but is only partially effective at checking reagent performance because the liquid control may require testing on a different type of test strip/cartridge than is used for whole blood. Some POCT instruments require the presence of erythrocytes to trigger the end-point detection system and lyophilised controls containing them are available but they are from anticoagulated blood [40]. The assigned ranges for some of these IQC materials is very wide, up to 2 INR units in some cases, rendering them almost ineffective unless users aim for narrower ranges either side of the target value. Electronic quality control is incorporated into POCT instruments. Self checks, such as temperature control, exist within the devices themselves. Some instruments can utilise an electronic control (EC) that takes the place of a test strip/cartridge and produces signals that test the optical and electronic systems by mimicking blood sample analysis. Whilst ingenious, EC alone checks analyser performance but not reagent performance and is not sufficient to use in isolation.

Laboratories should also be registered with an external quality assurance agency, such as the highly successful National External Quality Assurance Service (NEQAS) for Blood Coagulation in the UK. Lyophilised plasmas are sent to participants who generate INR results that are returned to UK NEQAS for retrospective statistical evaluation of each laboratory's performance in comparison with others throughout the UK. The UK NEQAS scheme provides a service for many more coagulation parameters than PT/INR and the surveys often reveal differences between alternative methods when measuring given analytes. In view of the nature of analysis by alternative local systems for analytes other than PT/INR, this is perhaps unsurprising. UK NEQAS adopts more than one model of survey analysis and will often demonstrate that although analysis of a given parameter via a specific methodology may deviate from the overall mean, sub-analysis shows that all, or at least most, users employing that methodology agree with each other within acceptable limits. This is not necessarily a clinical problem if methodology specific reference ranges are applied as all patients results will be relative to that range for that method.

Conversely, this should not be the case for INRs because the system is designed to significantly minimise result variation irrespective of locally employed systems. Surveys from UK NEQAS do however reveal differences between centres that suggest there are still standardisation issues with the INR system. Adoption of local system ISI assignment in recent years has improved laboratory agreement [21] yet it is still not a ubiquitous practice and variation continues to be apparent. A variety of factors further contribute to INR variability and we will now turn our attention to those issues.

FACTORS CONTRIBUTING TO INTER-LABORATORY INR VARIABILITY

Local system ISI corrects for major differences in PT/INR results between systems providing that the calibration is undertaken effectively. A number of variables can adversely impact on successful calibration:

- Calibration against an inappropriate IRP
- Insufficient normal and abnormal samples
- The abnormal samples used in a calibration must be distributed within the 2.0 – 4.5 range of INRs and have sufficient numbers of low, medium and high values. This is difficult to control when purchasing commercially prepared pools although unlikely to be a problem if manufacturers use the recommended numbers and spread of donors.
- Calculation errors
- Unrecognised analyser faults
- Operator training/variability, particularly for manual and semi-manual techniques
- Not using GMNPT or errors in generation of GMNPT i.e. unrepresentative donor population, technical faults, complications in pre-analytical variables

Even if an effective calibration is undertaken, performance of PTs in the diagnostic/monitoring setting is subject to the effects of pre-analytical variables, which themselves will impact on ISI generation if the samples used for calibration are thus affected.

Tri-sodium citrate is the anticoagulant of choice for venous blood samples requiring PT analysis because its removal of calcium ions can be overcome by test reagent calcium. One drawback is that it is a liquid anticoagulant with the potential for dilution-induced analytical error. Standard practice is for nine volumes of blood to be decalcified with one volume of anticoagulant - standardisation/calibration techniques and reference ranges are generated on the basis that this is the case for all samples. Underfilled samples can result in dilution of the clotting factors being assessed and lead to elevation of clotting times and erroneously high INRs, overfilled samples having the reverse effect. In patients with uncompromised coagulation, the in-built reserve coagulation capacity is often sufficient to generate a normal result unless the dilution is marked. This is, of course, not the case with orally anticoagulated patients and the dilution effect of an underfilled sample can markedly elevate the INR result and lead to unwarranted dose alterations. The prolongation of clotting times can be exacerbated by the relative excess of anticoagulant that may subsequently neutralise the calcium in the test reagent. Use of evacuated tubes should reduce the frequency of inappropriately filled tubes although there are occasions when the lids are removed and traditional syringe phlebotomy is applied, such as for collapsible veins. An interesting adjunct to this issue is that evacuated tubes can lose their vacuum in high-altitude areas due to reduced pressure between the tube and surrounding atmosphere and lead to unwitting underfilling.

Patients with haematocrits outside the range of 0.370 - 0.500 L/L will lead to relative increase or decrease of citrate concentration in the plasma and have similar effects to over or under-filling. These effects can be negated by adjusting the volume of citrate used (in a subsequent sample) by applying one of a number of available formulas such as the example below:

$$\frac{(100 - \text{haematocrit as a percentage}) \times \text{blood draw volume in mL}}{(595 - \text{haematocrit as a percentage})} = \text{volume of citrate required (mL)}$$

The citrate concentration itself inevitably impacts on clotting times, which become longer as the concentration increases [41]. Most laboratories employ concentrations between 0.105 – 0.109 mol/L (3.13 – 3.2%) although concentrations as high as 0.129 mol/L (3.8%) have been used. Plasmas used in ISI calibration should have been anticoagulated with the same citrate concentration as that used for local PT testing otherwise the results are not comparable.

Blood samples must be taken into plastic or non-wettable, siliconised glass collection tubes to prevent activation of contact factors. The citrate should have a pH no lower than 5 and ideally be buffered to provide a stable environment for clotting factors, some of which are labile. Some reports state that citrated blood samples for INR testing are stable for up to 24 hours at room temperature [42]. WHO recommend immediate centrifugation upon receipt and no later than 2 hours after blood collection. If analysis is to be delayed, the plasma should be removed with a plastic pipette and stored in a narrow, stoppered tube at room temperature and tested no later than 5 hours after blood collection. Good phlebotomy with a non-traumatic clean draw is essential to prevent activation, haemolysis and clotting.

The issues of unrecognised analyser faults, operator training/variability and GMNPT errors that affect ISI calibration equally affect day-to-day performance of PTs.

Patients requiring immediate anticoagulation may be given unfractionated heparin (UFH) therapy until the oral anticoagulant effect has reached an INR within the target therapeutic range. Care must be exercised when interpreting the INR result because the presence of UFH in the sample may further prolong the PT and give a false impression of the level of oral anticoagulation. In practice, therapeutic levels of UFH rarely interfere with PT analysis because of the powerful stimulus of a significant excess of tissue factor in thromboplastin reagents. Additionally, some manufacturers add heparin neutralisers to thromboplastin reagents to further reduce the likelihood of UFH interference, although they are only effective up to certain concentrations of UFH. Problems can also be encountered when blood samples are taken from central lines that have not been flushed sufficiently to prevent UFH entering the sample. Oral anticoagulant therapy inevitably affects APTT results but to a lesser extent than PT results. In the APTT there are more stages involving non-vitamin K dependent factors and they proceed at normal velocity, thereby rendering the APTT less sensitive as a monitoring tool. The APTT is commonly used for monitoring UFH therapy and the anticoagulant effect of UFH may be overestimated if the patient is also receiving oral anticoagulants.

Lupus anticoagulants (LA) present particular problems because their innate heterogeneity, which can vary over time even in individual patients, means that there is no specific pattern of standard coagulation screening results that can be ascribed. Classically, LA present as an isolated, elevated APTT, yet the marked variation in sensitivity to LA between routine APTT reagents means that not all LA will manifest in this way. It is rare for LA to prolong a PT because thromboplastins contain concentrated phospholipids that swamp most LA although there are occasions where both PT and APTT are elevated, and more rarely, only the PT is prolonged [43]. Some LA will not prolong the PT or APTT of a specific reagent pair and more sensitive assays are required for their detection. Patients with clinically significant PT-reacting LA present monitoring difficulties when treated with oral anticoagulant therapy because there is an ever-present risk of over-estimation of anticoagulation [44]. A patient whose LA prolongs the PT in routine diagnostic/monitoring use should be monitored with a different thromboplastin that is unaffected by that patient's LA. Antibody heterogeneity and reagent variability make this a feasible option for most patients. Alternative monitoring strategies are required where this is unachievable and measurement of factor II and factor X levels by one-stage clotting assays, where plasma (and LA) are diluted, has been used successfully. For patients with LA that overcome even the dilution effect, chromogenic factor X assays are available. A factor X level around 40% of normal equates to an INR of 2, and a level around 15% equates to an INR of 3.

Chapter 3

CLINICAL CONSIDERATIONS

Each clinic, hospital or healthcare provider involved in warfarin therapy should determine the best model of care or combinations thereof that suits their particular needs and population. In particular, guidelines for initiation/loading, dose maintenance, patient management, over-anticoagulation with or without bleeding and "bridging" should be established. Reference to established guidelines including but not limited to ACCP American College of Chest Physicians 8th edition (www.chestnet.org) [45], BSH British Society of Haematology (www.bcshguidelines.com) [46] and SIGN Scottish Intercollegiate Guidelines Network (www.sign.ac.uk) [47,48] should be made.

Warfarin is the most widely used oral anticoagulant in the UK although other oral anticoagulants are available which are commonly used in Euorope. These include the other 4-hydroxycoumarins, acenocoumarol and phenprocoumon. Acenocoumarol has a shorter half-life than warfarin whereas that of phenprocoumon is longer and both are not completely interchangeable with warfarin [49]. The relationship between the maintenance dose of warfarin, acenocoumarol and phenprocoumon is well established, whereas the relationship between warfarin and phenindione less so. In our clinic we use the guide given below in Table 1. The values between warfarin and phenindione are extrapolated using maintenance doses of warfarin and phenindione of 3mg to 9mg and 50mg to 150mgs respectively.

Superwarfarins are potent, highly lipophilic 4-hydroxycoumarin '2nd generation' derivatives and like warfarin they exert their anticoagulant effect by inhibiting the vitamin K epoxide reductase enzyme complex that recycles vitamin K 2,3-epoxide to vitamin K hydroquinone.

Table 1. Relationship between doses for 4-hydroxycoumarins

Dosage Conversions – Warfarin/Acenocoumarol/Phenindione		
Warfarin Dose	Acenocoumarol Dose	Phenindione Dose (fitted to available tablet strength)
1mg	0.5mg	≈ 20mg
2mg	1.0mg	≈ 35mg
3mg	1.5mg	50mg
4mg	2.0mg	≈ 70mg
5mg	2.5mg	≈ 80mg
6mg	3.0mg	100mg
7mg	3.5mg	≈ 120mg
8mg	4.0mg	≈ 135mg
9mg	4.5mg	150mg
10mg	5.0mg	≈170mg

Acenocoumarol 1mg is equivalent to Warfarin 1.5 - 2mg.
Phenindione 50mg is equivalent to Warfarin 3mg.
Reproduced with permission from the Centre for Haemostasis and Thrombosis, Guy's and St. Thomas' NHS foundation Trust, London, UK.

These compounds were developed to control populations of rodents that had developed resistance to warfarin. Commonly available superwarfarin compounds include difenacoum (Figure 8a), brodifacoum (Figure 8b), coumatetralyl and bromadialone. The extreme potency of these compounds precludes any clinical application.

The 1,3-indandiones e.g. phenindione (Figure 8c), are another group of vitamin K antagonists that exert their anticoagulant effect through inhibition of the VKORC. They were first identified by Kabat *et al* in 1944 as 2-substituted-1,3-indandiones [50]. These compounds have some commercial use as rodenticides but their hepatic toxicity prevents widespread clinical use [51].

It may be of interest to the reader that during investigations into the structural requirements for vitamin K activity, Lowenthal *et al* found that substitution of the 2-methyl group of vitamin K with a chlorine atom to form 2-chloro-3-phytyl-1,4-naphthoquinone (Figure 8d), or a bromine atom to form 2-bromo-3-phytyl-1,4-naphthoquinone conferred potent vitamin K antagonist properties [52]. The chlorine substituted compound, commonly referred to as "Chloro-K", has the greatest anticoagulant activity, producing its effect through inhibition of the γ-glutamyl carboxylase [53].

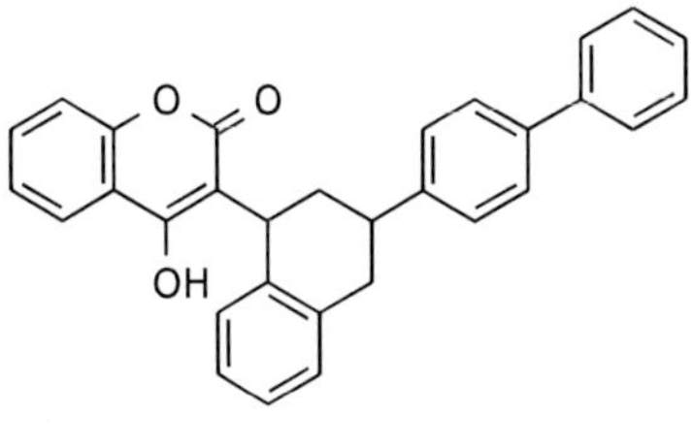

(a) Difenacoum

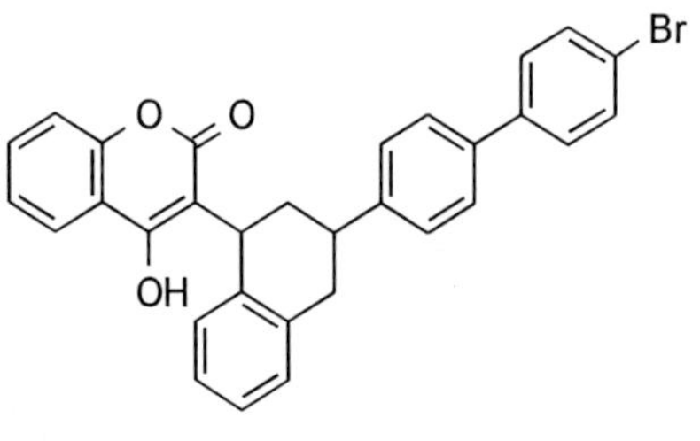

(b) Brodifacoum

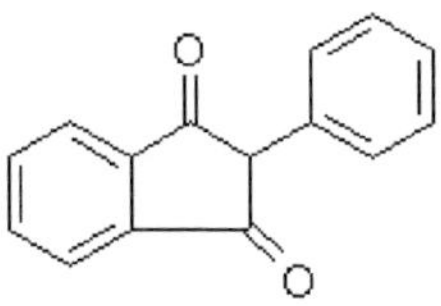

(c) Phenindione

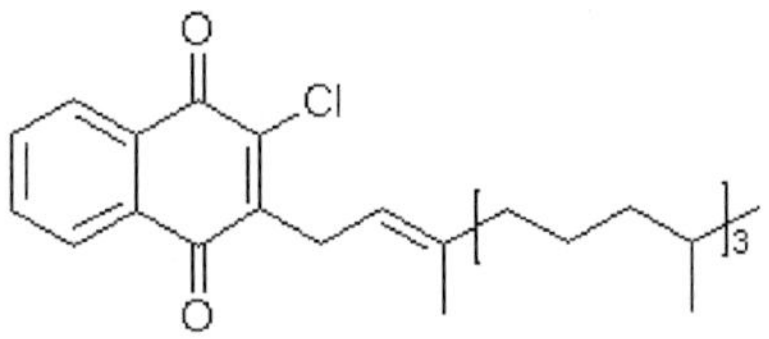

(d) 2-chloro-3-phytyl-1,4-naphthoquinone (Chloro-K)

Figure 8. Structural formulae of vitamin K antagonists not suggested for clinical use.

Vitamin E quinone has also been demonstrated as a vitamin K antagonist although the mechanism has yet to be defined conclusively [54]. Currently it is thought that this antagonism is a consequence of inhibition of CO_2 uptake and/or possibly interaction with essential thiol groups at the active site [55].

Two further series of compounds with little structural similarity to vitamin K also reportedly act as vitamin K antagonists. 2,3,5,6-Tetrachloro-4-pyridinol has anticoagulant activity [56,57] that is thought to originate from direct antagonism of γ-glutamyl carboxylase [58]. 6-Substituted imidazole (4,5-*b*) pyrimidines e.g. 6-chloro-2-trifluoromethyl-imidszo (4,5-*b*) pyrimidine exerts an anticoagulant probably through inhibition of the VKORC [59].

When introduced the oral anticoagulant ximelagatran (Exanta), a direct thrombin inhibitor, was expected to replace warfarin. However when reports of hepatotoxicity were becoming apparent its manufacturer had to withdraw it from further development.

At present other drugs offering the efficacy of warfarin without a need for monitoring, such as dabigatran (Pradaxa®) and rivaroxaban (Xarelto®), are becoming available and they will necessitate further review and changes in how we manage our clinics and treat our patients [60]. A comparison between the main features of warfarin, dabigatran and rivaroxaban is presented in Table 2.

Table 2. Comparison of new oral anticoagulants compared to warfarin

Feature	Warfarin	Dabigatran	Rivaroxaban
Site of action	VKORC	Thrombin	FXa
Immediate/delayed anticoagulation	Delayed	Immediate	Immediate
Requires laboratory monitoring	Yes (PT/INR)	No	No
Dosing	Variable	Fixed dose	Fixed dose
Can be used in pregnancy	No	No	No
Available antidote	Yes	No	No
Half-life	2.5 days	14 – 17 h	5 – 13 h
Mode(s) of elimination	92% renal	80% renal 20% biliary	66% renal 33% biliary
Plasma protein binding	99.5%	25 – 30%	90%
Bioavailability	100%	5%	>80%

PT, prothrombin time; INR, international normalized ratio; VKORC; vitamin K epoxide reductase complex; FXa, activated factor X.

Although the new oral anticoagulants are more expensive than warfarin, this could be at least partly offset by the reduction in clinical complications such as heart attacks, and reduction in monitoring costs [61].

Safety

The NPSA (National Patient Safety Agency) Alert 18 from 2008, "Actions that can make anticoagulant therapy safer" www.npsa.nhs.uk/nrls/alerts-and-directives/alerts/anticoagulant will be important in any future management structure for anticoagulation clinics and the professionals involved with these. To quote:

> "Anticoagulants are one of the classes of medicines most frequently identified as causing preventable harms and admissions to hospitals. The NPSA has produced the following patient safety alert and support materials to help manage the risks associated with anticoagulants and reduce the risks of patients being harmed in the future"

Numerous documents are provided for guidance on use of anticoagulants with a view to assisting healthcare practitioners in achieving the aims of the alert, which are detailed in Table 3.

Table 3. Aims of the National Patient Safety Alert 18 (2008)

Healthcare organisations in England and Wales should:
• Ensure staff are properly trained. • Review and / or update written procedures and clinical protocols to ensure they reflect safe practice. • Audit anticoagulant services using British Society for Haematology/NPSA safety indicators as part of the annual medicines management audit programme. • Ensure that patients prescribed anticoagulants receive appropriate information. • Promote safe practice for prescribers and pharmacists to check that patients' blood clotting (INR) is monitored regularly and that the INR level is safe before issuing or dispensing repeat prescriptions for oral anticoagulants. • Promote safe practice for prescribers co-prescribing one or more clinically significant interacting medicines for patients already on oral anticoagulants: arrange for additional INR blood tests and inform the anticoagulant service that an interacting medicine has been prescribed. • Ensure dental practitioners manage patients on anticoagulants according to evidence-based therapeutic guidelines. • Amend local policies to standardise the range of anticoagulant products used, incorporating characteristics which promote safer use. • Promote the use of written safe practice procedures for the administration of anticoagulants in social care settings.

With patient safety as the number one objective clinics should periodically audit their results and review exceptional cases. Between 50% and 75% of INRs should ideally be within the designated therapeutic range.

ADVERSE EFFECTS

Despite its effectiveness, treatment with warfarin has several shortcomings including interactions with many commonly used medications and some foods, requirement of frequent monitoring with blood tests [62], and it has a narrow therapeutic range which requires expert dose management. As such it is one of the most quoted medications for adverse event and drug error reporting. There are a number of recognised adverse effects associated with warfarin therapy.

Hemorrhage and Reversal of Over Anticoagulation

The intensity of anticoagulation, the concomitant use of agents that interfere with haemostasis, the length of therapy and patient characteristics are major determinants of warfarin-induced bleeding [63]. Risk factors including old age, serious illness, cerebral, cardiac, kidney or liver disease, cerebro vascular or peripheral vascular disease, and an unstable INR can contribute to major bleeding which has been reported in 1.1% to 8.1% of patients during each year of long-term treatment.

Numerous experimental and observational studies have attempted to estimate the incidence of major haemorrhage for patients receiving warfarin therapy [64-73].

This bleeding risk can be further increased when treatment is combined with drugs such as clopidogrel, aspirin, or other non-steroidal anti-inflammatory drugs which demonstrate an anti-platelet effect [74] as well as with alcohol abuse. It is more common within the first three months of treatment and is often secondary to trauma, but can indicate an underlying undiagnosed comorbidity [75]. The risk of bleeding should be evaluated and discussed with each patient before anticoagulation is initiated [76].

The age of the patient alone should not be a contraindication to treatment with warfarin. Some reports suggest that for each decade above the age of 40 this raises the risk of major bleeding by almost 50% reaching its maximum effect above 70 years [77], whereas others have found that there is no difference with age below 70 years [75].

There are conflicting studies on whether age is an independent risk factor for bleeding and old age is not in itself a contraindication to warfarin so patients' characteristics should be assessed.

For example:

- the risk of falls and possible causes
- poor nutrition which might result in a relative deficiency of vitamin K and increased sensitivity to warfarin
- hypertension
- cerebrovascular disease

- serious heart disease
- renal insufficiency
- malignancy

However, age is a risk factor for the prothrombin time to be more unstable. There is a 15% increase in the risk of anticoagulation having to be interrupted because of a raised INR with every 10 year increase in age [78].

Whether bleeding is expressed as an absolute risk per annum or as a relative risk the INR is the most important factor. It has been suggested that the bleeding rate is doubled as the INR increases from 2.0-2.9 to 3.0-4.4, four times between 4.5-6.0, and was multiplied by five times when the INR is above 7.0 [79].

The only common side effect of warfarin is bleeding and although the risk is small it is definite. Any new diagnosis, treatment or major change in the patient's condition, especially in the presence of poor diet, requires further assessment of the risks and benefits of continuing oral anticoagulation [80].

Therefore a risk benefit analysis for each patient is necessary to establish that any benefits outweigh the risks. Any symptoms including haemoptysis, excessive bruising, bleeding from the nose or gums, or blood in urine or stool should be taken seriously even if they are thought to have a simple origin as they may indicate being over-anticoagulated due to interactions or accidental or deliberate overdosing.

Any INR above 5.0 requires close monitoring and depending if there are signs of bleeding or not, may require intervention. When the INR is <7 and there are no signs of bleeding, withholding warfarin should be sufficient. 1 to 2 mg of oral vitamin K_1 reduces the INR in the range 5.0 to 10.0 to 2.0 to 5.0 within 24-48 hours and this together with withholding the warfarin should be sufficient in the absence of bleeding for an INR of 7 or greater. Any INR of 7 or greater with signs of non-life threatening bleeding should be treated with a Prothrombin Complex Concentrate (PCC) 500iu, vitamin K_1 and withholding warfarin. PCCs contain the four vitamin K-dependent coagulation factors (II, VII, IX and X), and the vitamin K-dependent naturally occurring inhibitors protein C and protein S, which are all human plasma derived. They correct clotting factor deficiencies faster and more completely than plasma and additionally reduce the risk of fluid overload, transmission of infectious agents and anaphylaxis. As the half life of warfarin is long, approximately 36 hours, careful monitoring should continue over several days because when the effects of vitamin K_1 wear off the INR may rebound. An INR should be performed immediately after PCC administration (< 1 h) and then at least daily [81]. This closer monitoring of the INR is essential both to detect the transient warfarin resistance caused by too much vitamin K_1, usually 5 to 10mg, and to avoid further over-anticoagulation. Life threatening bleeding or an intracranial bleed should be treated with full dose PCC (25 to 50 iu/Kg) and 10mg vitamin K i.v. with careful monitoring and repeated doses as necessary.

Bleeding or an unstable dose-response is a trigger to review the need for continued warfarin treatment, which ideally should be reviewed at regular intervals in all patients. The overanticoagulation and reversal procedure employed in the authors' institution is outlined below.

Overanticoagulation and Reversal Procedure

For venous INR levels between 5.0 and 7.0 (refer to maintenance dose adjustment tables – see p49 - 53)

Any INR >10.0 must be discussed with a Haematologist.

If there is any suspicion of life threatening bleed, i.e. intracerebral or intracavity bleed, call resuscitation team immediately for support and transfer to Accident and Emergency Department.

Moderate Overdose: INR >7 -10

Without signs of bleeding

- Omit oral anticoagulant dose on that day
- Administer Vitamin K 1mg orally for all patients.
- Recheck INR the following day

With signs of bleeding

- Omit oral anticoagulant on that day
- Obtain recent bleeding history e.g. incidence of epistaxis, haematuria, malaena
- Give PCC. For dosing advice, contact Haematologist.
- Give Vitamin K 1mg orally.
- Carry out FBC to determine evidence of blood loss, when directed.
- Recheck INR the following day

Severe Overdosage: INR>10

With or without bleeding

- Omit oral anticoagulant for minimum of two days
- Give PCC. For dosing advice, contact Haematologist.
- Give Vitamin K 2mg orally.
- Contact Haematologist who will consider whether the patient requires admission depending on the clinical circumstances and risk of haemorrhage. The total number of days to miss anticoagulant will also be advised at this point, as will the new dose of warfarin to restart once the result is back within the patient's therapeutic range.
- Recheck the INR 20 minutes after administration of PCC. If the INR is within range, bring the patient back the next day for another INR check. Do not restart the warfarin at this point. If the INR is still higher than the therapeutic range, discuss the case with the Haematologist.

Post-Reversal INR Values

Post reversal INR values should lie within or below the patient's therapeutic range the following day.

Patients Experiencing INR 7-10

- The patient can resume their usual dose if there was no reason for the high result or the causative factor has been removed, and the INR is within range.
- If the INR is below range, a loading dose should be given according to the dosage tables.
- If there is an ongoing reason for the high result, e.g. patient is continuing to drink despite warnings/amiodarone has been commenced, the dose should be reduced as per protocol.

Patients Experiencing INR >10

Each patient who experiences an INR >10 must be discussed with a Haemophilia Physician prior to resuming the maintenance dose.

(Procedure reproduced with permission from the Centre for Haemostasis and Thrombosis, Guy's and St. Thomas' NHS foundation Trust, London, UK)

Warfarin Necrosis

Warfarin necrosis is a rare complication which frequently occurs shortly after commencing treatment in patients with protein C deficiency [82]. During initial treatment protein C levels decrease faster than the other factors due to it's relatively shorter half-life, which paradoxically increase the blood's tendency to coagulate. This can result in thrombosis with skin necrosis and gangrene of limbs. In children who are homozygous for certain protein C mutations "Purpura Fulminans" can be observed [83].

Osteoporosis

There are conflicting reports that warfarin can reduce bone mineral density resulting in osteoporosis-related fractures. In 2006 a retrospective study of 14,564 Medicare recipients there was a 60% increased risk of osteoporosis-related fractures in men but not in women when on warfarin for more than one year. The mechanism for this is unknown but it was thought to be either reduced intake of vitamin K, which is necessary for bone health, or interference in the carboxylation of extra-hepatic vitamin K-dependent proteins (osteocalcin) by warfarin [84].

Vascular and Aortic Calcification

The extra hepatic vitamin K-dependent protein Matrix-Gla Protein (MGP) protects against vascular calcification. Warfarin therapy prevents the production of active MGP leading to the possibility that long term exposure to vitamin K antagonists could lead to inappropriate calcification of tissue. Active MGP has been shown to be compromised in patients with calcific aortic valve disease possibly as a consequence of a decrease in the local expression of MGP [85].

Purple Toe Syndrome

Commonly within 3 to 8 weeks of starting treatment, another rare complication can be observed - “purple toe syndrome”. This aetiology is thought to result from cholesterol crystal emboli being released into the blood vessels of the skin as a result of warfarin-induced bleeding into atherosclerotic plaques, with subsequent occlusion of dermal arterioles and ischemic infarction of the epidermis [86]. Another theory postulates that warfarin may cause cholesterol embolisation by contributing to the gradual loss of a protective fibrin layer overlying an ulcerated atherosclerotic plaque [86]. Typically the big toe is affected but other parts of the feet can be involved including the plantar surface.

As shown in Figure 9, a blueish purple area is noted which may be painful and treatment may have to be discontinued [87]. The discoloration usually blanches with pressure but fades when the legs are not in a dependent position [87]. The purple colour fluctuates in intensity but persists indefinitely, even if warfarin therapy is discontinued, although the toe pain will resolve. INR is within the therapeutic range and the pulse in the distal lower extremity is normal.

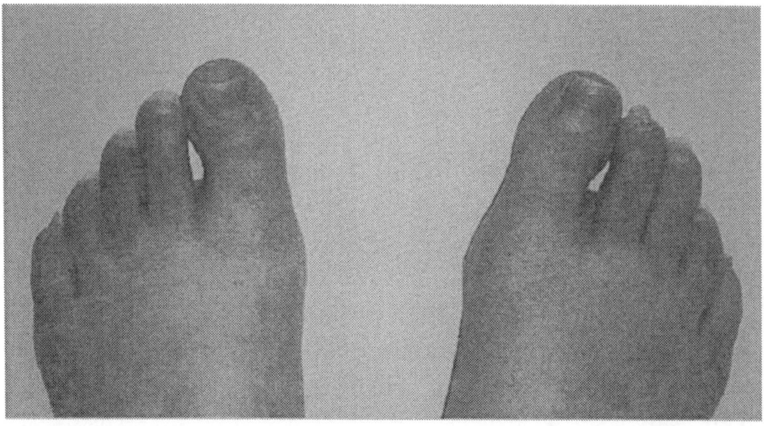

Figure 9. Purple toe syndrome (reproduced with permission from Dr Savita Rangarajan).

The diagnosis can be confirmed histologically by tissue biopsy of the affected skin, which reveals pathognomic needle shaped clefts in the arterioles. Anticoagulation and thrombolysis are contraindicated. Associated risk factors such as hypertension, hypercholesterolaemia and smoking should be managed aggressively [88].

Drug Interactions

As there is great variation in the metabolism of warfarin between patients and considering its interaction with commonly used medicines together with some foods [89], finding the correct dosage can be extremely difficult and in turn illustrates the need for careful monitoring. When a medication that is known to interact with warfarin is started, stopped or the dose adjusted then an INR check after 2-3 days is justified and the warfarin dose increased or decreased until a new ideal dosage is found. The main mechanisms of drug interactions with warfarin are:

- Reduced vitamin K synthesis by gut flora
- Altered metabolism of warfarin
- Direct interference of vitamin K cycle
- Reduced platelet function
- Direct gastrointestinal injury

By reducing the metabolism of warfarin, antibiotics such as metronidazole or the macrolides (azithromycin, clarithromycin, erythromycin, and roxithromycin) can increase its effect [90]. Other broad-spectrum antibiotics will reduce the normal gut bacteria, which make significant amounts of vitamin K, and exert a similar effect [91]. Rifampin however induces the cytochrome P450 (CYP) system and reduces the effect of warfarin. Antifungals such as fluconazole and miconazole increase the effect of warfarin by inhibition of the CYP system, as does amiodarone. Selective serotonin re-uptake inhibitor antidepressants can enhance warfarin anticoagulation by impairing platelet aggregation and inhibition of CYP. Anti-inflammatory agents erode the protective lining of the stomach thereby promoting gastro-intestinal bleeding, and additionally decrease platelet function, which is of course the mechanism of the antiplatelet drugs such as aspirin and clopidogrel. Excessive alcohol is also known to affect the metabolism of warfarin and increase the INR. In contrast, foods or products containing large amounts of vitamin K will decrease its effect.

Alcohol consumption and its interaction with warfarin therapy is complex. A review article [92] concluded:

1. Intermediate use (2-3 drinks per day) probably does not alter the INR at all.
2. Intermittent large amount of alcohol drinking leads to an increase in INR, because the alcohol interferes with warfarin metabolism, i.e. warfarin is metabolized less rapidly.
3. Chronic heavy alcohol intake results in a decreased INR, because the alcohol actually increases the metabolism of warfarin.

Alcohol is broken down to acetaldehyde in the liver predominantly by either alcohol dehydrogenase (ADH) or the CYP system [93]. In the absence of alcohol, CYP enzymes break down warfarin (and other drugs) and the resulting metabolites are excreted. Intermittent intake of large amounts will increase INR because CYP is required to metabolise alcohol as well as warfarin, so warfarin metabolism is reduced due to competition for CYP between alcohol and warfarin resulting in higher warfarin levels in the body. Intermediate alcohol intake (2-3 drinks/day) however is unlikely to alter the degree of anticoagulation. Conversely, in chronic heavy drinkers who are sober, CYP activity is enhanced so warfarin breakdown is increased, resulting in reduced levels in the body and a decrease in INR. In an intoxicated chronic heavy drinker, although CYP activity is enhanced, most of it is involved in alcohol metabolism so warfarin metabolism is reduced and can result in an increase in INR. Levels of the main CYP enzyme for alcohol metabolism, CYP2E1, vary between individuals, so in those with low CYP2E1 activity the potential for alcohol-warfarin interactions increases because of the shift of other CYP enzymes for alcohol metabolism [94].

Alcohol can also impair platelet function, mainly by inhibiting platelet phospholipase 2 and thus reducing formation of thromboxane A2, an important *in vivo* platelet activator [95]. Red wine is rich in polyphenolic compounds which further enhance its affect on platelet function by reducing prostanoid synthesis from arachidonate, reducing platelet activity mediated by nitric oxide and increasing vitamin E levels while decreasing oxidation of platelets submitted to oxidative stress. Interestingly, the rebound phenomenon of platelet hyperaggregability observed after acute alcohol consumption is not seen with wine consumption [96]. Alcohol can also cause thrombocytopenia resulting from a direct toxic effect on platelet production and survival.

Thyroid function appears to be important in warfarin dosing with hypothyroidism rendering patients less responsive [97] and hyperthyroidism rendering patients more responsive [98]. Decreased catabolism of the vitamin K dependent factors is thought to be the cause of the decreased response in hypothyroidism [99].

The increased sensitivity associated with hyperthyroidism may be due to the high levels of thyroxine increasing the affinity of warfarin for receptor sites in the liver with a consequent decrease in production of vitamin K dependent factors. Increased catabolism of vitamin K dependent factors may also contribute.

Numerous other drugs and foodstuffs have been associated with warfarin interactions, such as acetaminophen which enhances the effect by direct interference with the vitamin K cycle, or carbamazepine, which reduces the warfarin effect by CYP induction.

Many herbs also react with warfarin (100), and ginger, garlic, ginseng, and ginkgo have been reported to increase bleeding and bruising in patients on warfarin, as have borage (starflower) oil (*Borago officinalis*)and fish oils [101]. St. John's Wort can result in a reduced anticoagulant effect by induction of CYP isoenzymes (102).

Crucial to maintaining stable control is consistent consumption, or no consumption, of foods with very high vitamin K content. The evidence for association is stronger for some drugs and foodstuffs than others, some being based on small numbers of cases studies or isolated cases. Table 4 lists drugs and foodstuffs reported to interact with warfarin and Appendix 1 outlines the clinical relevance for those most commonly encountered.

In general, considering the number of substances that interact with warfarin a detailed history of all medication, including over the counter products is essential when considering warfarin resistance, difficult to control patients or initiating therapy. Importantly, we should be open to new associations and possible interactions.

In the UK, between 2003 and 2004, The Committee on Safety of Medicines received numerous reports of a possible interaction between patients taking cranberry juice and an increase in INR, possibly due to CYP inhibition, and hence risk of haemorrhage [103].

Table 4. Drugs and foodstuffs reported to have interactions with warfarin

	Increased anticoagulant effect		**Decreased anticoagulant effect**
Drugs	Acarbose	Leflunomide	Azathioprine
	Acetaminophen	Levamisole	Barbiturates
	Acetylsalicylic acid	Levofloxacin	Bosentan
	Amiodarone	Lovastatin	Candesartan cilexetil
	Amoxicillin	Metolazone	Carbamazepine
	Anabolic steroids	Metronidazole	Chelation therapy with EDTA
	Azithromycin	Miconazole	Chlordiazepoxide
	Celecoxib	Nalidixic acid	Cholestyramine
	Chloramphenicol	Norfloxacin	Cyclosporine
	Choral hydrate	Ofloxacin	Dicloxacillin
	Cimetidine	Orlistat	Etodolac
	Ciprofloxacin	Omeprazole	Etretinate
	Citalopram	Paclitaxel	Griseofulvin
	Clarithromycin	Paracetamol	Influenza vaccine
	Clofibrate	Phenylbutazone	Mercaptopurine
	CMF	Phenytoin	Mesalamine
	Cotrimoxazole	Piroxicam	Naficillin
	Curbicin	Propafenone	Raloxifene hydrochoride
	Danazol	Propoxyphene	Ribavirin
	Danshen/methyl salicylate	Propranolol	Rifampin
	Dextropropoxyphen	Quinidine	Ritonavir
	Diltiazem	Ritonavir	Sucralfate
	Disopyramide	Rofecoxib	Sulfasalazine
	Disulfiram	Ropinirole	Telmisartan
	Entacapone	Saquinavir	Terbinafine
	Erythromycin	Sertraline	Trazodone
	Felbamate	Simvastatin	Ubidicarenone
	Fenofibrate	Sulfinpyrazone	Vitamin K
	Fluconazole	Sulindac	
	Fluorouracil	Sulindac	
	Fluvastatin	Tamoxifen	
	Fluvoxamine	Terbinafine	
	Gatifloxacin	Tetracycline	
	Gemcitabine	Ticlopidine	
	Gemfibrozil	Tolmetin	
	Ifosphamide	Tolterodine	
	Indomethacin	Tramadol	
	Interferon	Trastuzumab	

Table 4. (Continued)

	Increased anticoagulant effect		Decreased anticoagulant effect
	Isoniazid	Troglitazone	
	Itraconazole	Voriconazole	
	Ketoconazole	Zileuton	
Foodstuffs	Alcohol (acute consumption)		Alcohol (chronic consumption)
	Bishop's weed		Avocado (high intake)
	Boldo-fenugreek		Chewing tobacco
	Cat's Claw		Co-enzyme Q10
	Chamomile		Ginseng (American & Oriental)
	Cranberry juice		Green tea
	Danshen		High vitamin K content foods
	Devil's Claw		Soy milk
	Dong quai		St. John's Wort
	Echinacea		Sushi containing seaweed
	Eucalyptus		Vitamin C (large doses)
	Feverfew		Yarrow
	Fish oil		
	Garlic		
	Ginger		
	Ginko biloba		
	Grapefruit juice		
	Kava		
	Liquorice		
	Lime		
	Lycium barbarum (Goji berry or Chinese wolfberry)		
	Mango		
	Papain (from papaya)		
	Quilinggao		
	Red clover		
	Vitamin E		
	Willow bark		

CMF; cyclophosphamide/methotrexate/fluorouracil, EDTA, ethylene diamine tetra-acetic acid. Data taken from Holbrook *et al* [89] & Nutescu *et al* [105].

A review in 2006 found no cases of this interaction reported to the FDA [104] and data establishing a causal relationship is still lacking. Nevertheless, many authors suggest that both doctors and patients be made aware of this possibility.

Contraindications for Warfarin Therapy in Pregnancy

As oral anticoagulants cross the placenta they should ideally be avoided throughout pregnancy but especially during the first and third trimesters [106,107]. Women of child bearing age should be counselled on the importance of this together with the fact that should they become pregnant then immediate advice should be obtained. A particularly risky period is between the sixth and twelfth weeks of gestation when a combination of birth defects can occur resulting in Foetal Warfarin Syndrome (FWS), (warfarin embryopathy, or coumarin embryopathy). FWS is characterized by calcified epiphyses (*chondrodysplasia punctata*) and a characteristic nasal hypoplasia (Figure 10), with the calcifications in the vertebral column, femur, and heel bone showing a peculiar stippled appearance on X-rays (Figure 11). Limb abnormalities, such as brachydactyly together with non-skeletal abnormalities such as low birth weight and developmental problems are also seen [108, 109].

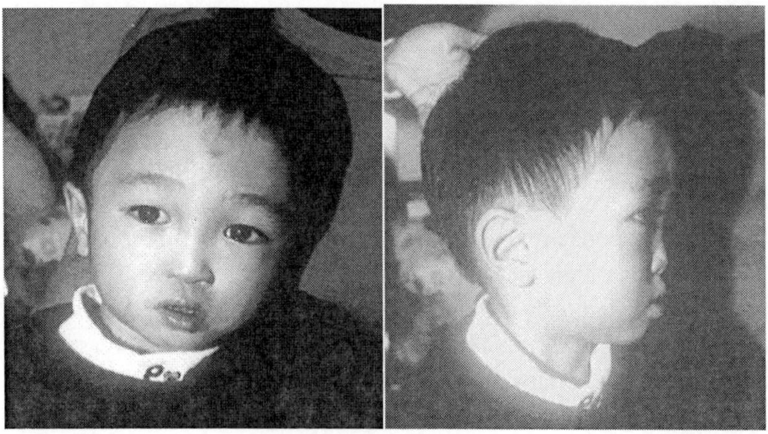

Figure 10. Hypoplasia of mid-face and nose in foetal warfarin syndrome. (Reproduced with permission from the Chang Gung Medical Journal; Hou J. Fetal Warfarin Syndrome. *Chang Gung Med J* 2004;9:691-695).

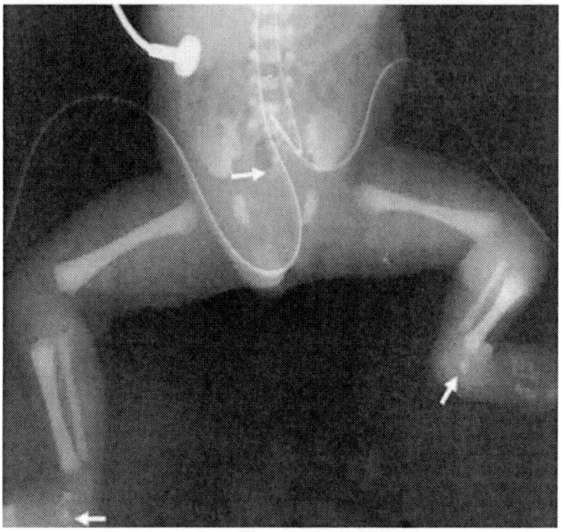

Figure 11. X-ray showing stippling in the sacral area and tarsal bones (arrowed) in foetal warfarin syndrome. (Reproduced with permission from the Chang Gung Medical Journal; Hou J. Fetal Warfarin Syndrome. *Chang Gung Med J* 2004;9:691-695).

The pathogenesis of FWS is probably from haemorrhage into any of several organs resulting from warfarin crossing the placenta and reaching significant levels in the foetal circulation [110].

In one report, almost 30% of children (10 of 35) born to mothers with a prosthetic heart valve were malformed if acenocoumarol was taken through the period covering 6-12 weeks gestation, but none of 19 developed a malformation when this drug was replaced with low molecular weight heparin before the sixth week [111]. Second and third trimesters birth defects are less common, and if they occur, differ greatly from FWS and are associated with central nervous system abnormalities, including microcephaly [108], spasticity, seizures, and eye defects [108,109]. Hence two distinct combinations of congenital abnormalities can arise depending upon when the exposure happens. As warfarin passes through the placental barrier it can cause foetal bleeding and is commonly associated with spontaneous abortion, stillbirth, neonatal death, and preterm birth [109]. However breastfeeding on warfarin is safe as there is minimal excretion into breast milk. [112].

Anticoagulation therefore poses a serious problem in pregnant women requiring treatment for vital indications, such as stroke prevention in those with artificial heart valves, and local guidelines for these patients should be established.

Chapter 4

DOSING AND MONITORING

LOADING

Warfarin is rapidly and completely absorbed and very few cases of "warfarin resistance" will be due to malabsorption. Its effect on the vitamin K-dependent factors II, VII, IX, X, protein C and protein S (and protein Z) is not uniform and care should be taken when determining that a patient is established in their therapeutic range.

The INR can be measured daily or every other day during loading with the dose of warfarin, which is usually taken in the evening titrated against that morning's INR result. It is then measured at increasing intervals depending on response.

For many a loading dose of 10 mg on both the first and second days is customary. However a reduced starting dose of 5 mg per day will achieve an INR of 2.0 in four to five days and may be safer in select groups of patients such as the elderly, impaired cardiac or liver function, ill or those with below average body weight. This together with the poorly-predictable pharmacokinetics of warfarin has lead to reports of several algorithms for commencing treatment:

1. The Kovacs 10 mg algorithm was better than a 5 mg algorithm [113].
2. The Fennerty 10 mg regimen is for urgent anticoagulation [114]. (Figure 12)
3. The Tait 5 mg regimen is for "routine" (low-risk) anticoagulation [115].

Day	UFH monitoring	INR (9 – 10 am)	Warfarin dose given at 5 pm (mg)
1	APTT ratio 1.5 – 2.5	-	0
2	APTT ratio 1.5 – 2.5	-	0
3	APTT ratio 1.5 – 2.5	<1.4	10
		<1.8	10
4	APTT ratio 1.5 – 2.5	1.8	1
		>1.8	0.5
		<2.0	10
		2.0 – 2.1	5
		2.2 – 2.3	4.5
		2.4 – 2.5	4
		2.6 – 2.7	3.5
		2.8 – 2.9	3
5	APTT ratio 1.5 – 2.5	3.0 – 3.1	2.5
	Stop UFH after dose on Day 5	3.2 – 3.3	2
		3.4	1.5
		3.5	1
		3.6 – 4.0	0.5
		>4.0	0
			Predicted maintenance dose:
		<1.4	>8
		1.4	8
		1.5	7.5
		1.6 – 1.7	7
		1.8	6.5
		1.9	6
		2.0 – 2.1	5.5
		2.2 – 2.3	5
6		2.4 – 2.6	4.5
		2.7 – 3.0	4
		3.1 – 3.5	3.5
		3.6 – 4.0	3
		4.1 – 4.5	Miss out next day's dose then give 2 mg
		>4.5	Miss out next day's dose then give 1 mg

(1) APTT ratio for UFH monitoring should be within or below therapeutic range (1.5-2.5). If APTT ratio is above this range the heparin effect on INR is neutralised with protamine (0.4µg/mL) plasma added to the sample.

(2) If heparin treatment is not being given, start the schedule at Day 3.

(3) Special care should be taken with patients with heart failure or liver disease and with those immediately after an operation as their sensitivity to warfarin may vary with time

(4) If INR on day 6 is <2..0 heparin may be given again until the INR is within the desired range

(5) If the INR on Day 3 is ≥1.4 the initial dose of warfarin should be reduced and the schedule is no longer relevant UFH, unfractionated heparin; APTT, activated partial thromboplastin time; INR, international normalised ratio.

Figure 12. Warfarin schedule for urgent anticoagulation. Adapted by permission from BMJ Publishing Group Ltd. (Fennerty A, Campbell IA, Routledge PA. Anticoagulants in venous thromboembolism. *BMJ* 1988; 297:1285 –1288).

The Fennerty regimen is widely used for standard warfarin initiation or urgent anticoagulation. Lenzini et al. derived and prospectively validated a model including CYP29C and VKORC1 genotypes [116]. This algorithm can be found at www.WarfarinDosing.org, a website programme with dosing calculators and other decision support tools for clinicians' use when initiating warfarin therapy.

ADJUSTING THE MAINTENANCE DOSE

Recommendations by many national bodies including the American College of Chest Physicians are helpful in managing dose adjustments [45,46,117]. Between individuals the daily maintenance dose can vary considerably but between 0.5 mg/day and 15 mg/day is usual and this can fluctuate over time. On average a dose of 4.5 mg/day is common but care should be taken in the elderly as this can be lower.

Once stable many patients can be controlled with 4-8 weekly testing and dose adjustment, but others will need more frequent assessment and some will need less. Although historically an empirical approach to warfarin dosing has been employed published dose-adjustment tables can help [118]. Dose adjustment tables used in the authors' institution are detailed below in Tables 5a-5h, reproduced with permission from the Centre for Haemostasis and Thrombosis, Guy's and St. Thomas' NHS foundation Trust, London, UK.

For Lower Therapeutic Range (INR 2.0 – 3.0)

Table 5a. Dose adjustments for lower therapeutic range (INR 2.0 - 3.0) when INR sub-therapeutic

Sub-therapeutic INR		Dose adjustment	Next Appointment
Slight	1.8 – 1.9	Stat loading dose for 1 day	As before, but max. 4 weeks
Moderate	1.5 – 1.7	Stat loading dose for 2 days	2-4 weeks
Significant	<1.5	Stat loading dose for 3 days	1 week 3-4 days if LMWH required

Table 5b. Dose adjustments for lower therapeutic range (INR 2.0 - 3.0) when over-anticoagulated

Over-anticoagulated		Dose adjustment	Next Appointment
Slight	3.1 - 3.3	Continue as before	As before, but max 4 weeks
Moderate	3.4 – 3.7	Omit dose for 1 day	2-4 weeks
Significant	3.8 - 4.5	Omit doses for 2 days	2 weeks
Significant	4.6 – 5.9	Omit doses for 2 days	1 week
Severe	6.0 - 7.0	Omit warfarin for 3 days	Next day
	>7.0	Omit warfarin and administer Vit K Follow 'Management of Over Anticoagulation' guideline	Next day

Evidence of bleeding may require a change in this schedule, or referral to a Haematologist, at any INR.

For Therapeutic Range (INR 2.5 – 3.0)

Table 5c. Dose adjustments for therapeutic range INR 2.5 - 3.0 when INR sub-therapeutic

Sub-therapeutic INR		Dose adjustment	Next Appointment
Slight	2.3 - 2.4	Continue same dose	As before, but max 4 weeks
Moderate	1.9 - 2.2	Stat loading dose for 1 day	2-4 weeks
Significant	1.5 - 1.8	Stat loading doses for 2 days	2 weeks
Severe	< 1.5	Stat loading doses for 3 days	1 week 4 days if LMWH required

As the effect of warfarin is subject to multiple interactions, rechecking the INR within a few days of any change in medication or clinical condition is essential. Multiple co-morbidities and a need for many other medications may increase the risk of an unstable anticoagulant response and starting or stopping therapy with other drugs, especially antibiotics and cardiac medications, changes in diet or bowel function can all influence the INR.

Table 5d. Dose adjustments for therapeutic range (INR 2.5 - 3.0) when over-anticoagulated

Over-anticoagulated		Dose adjustment	Next Appointment
Slight	3.1 - 3.3	Continue as before	As before, but max 4 weeks
Moderate	3.4 – 3.7	Omit dose for 1 day	2-4 weeks
Significant	3.8 - 4.5	Omit doses for 2 days	2 weeks
Significant	4.6 – 5.9	Omit doses for 2 days	1 week
Severe	6.0 - 7.0	Omit warfarin for 3 days	Next day
	>7.0	Omit warfarin and administer Vit K Follow 'Management of Over Anticoagulation' guideline	Next day

Evidence of bleeding may require a change in this schedule, or referral to a Haematologist, at any INR

For Intermediate Therapeutic Range (INR 2.5 – 3.5)

Table 5e. Dose adjustments for intermediate therapeutic range (INR 2.5 - 3.5) when INR sub-therapeutic

Sub-therapeutic INR		Dose adjustment	Next Appointment
Slight	2.3 - 2.4	Continue same dose	As before, but max 4 weeks
Moderate	1.9 - 2.2	Stat loading dose for 1 day	2-4 weeks
Significant	1.5 - 1.8	Stat loading doses for 2 days	2 weeks
Severe	< 1.5	Stat loading doses for 3 days	1 week 4days if LMWH required

Warfarin therapy is a partnership between patient and clinician to keep the INR within a therapeutic range. To be successful it will require regular monitoring and considerable effort to educate patients about how warfarin works, why their dose requirement may change, and the likely settings and symptoms of bleeding complications. The ultimate aim of this is patient safety by minimising both the bleeding risk associated with a high INR and the risks associated with a low INR.

Table 5f. Dose adjustments for intermediate therapeutic range (INR 2.5 - 3.5) when over-anticoagulated

Over-anticoagulated		**Dose Adjustment**	**Next Appointment**
Slight	3.6 - 3.8	Continue as before	As before but max 4 weeks
Moderate	3.9 – 4.2	Omit dose for 1 day	Half previous interval
Significant	4.3 - 5.0	Omit dose for 2 days	2 weeks
Significant	5.1 - 5.9	Omit dose for 2 days	1 week
Severe	6.0-7.0	Omit warfarin for 3 days	
	>7.0	Omit warfarin and administer Vit K Follow 'Management of Over Anticoagulation' guideline	

Evidence of bleeding may require a change in this schedule, or referral to a Haematologist, at any INR.

For Upper Therapeutic Range (INR 3.0 – 4.0)

Table 5g. Dose adjustments for upper therapeutic range (INR 3.0 – 4.0) when INR sub-therapeutic

Sub-therapeutic INR		**Dose Adjustment**	**Next Appointment**
Slight	2.8 - 2.9	Continue as before	As before, but max 4 weeks
Moderate	2.3 - 2.7	Stat loading dose for 1 day	2-4 weeks
Significant	1.5 - 2.2	Stat loading doses for 2 days	2 weeks
Severe	<1.5	Stat loading doses for 3 days	1 week 4 days if LMWH required

In recent years bespoke as well as commercially available computer assisted dosing software packages have transformed the record keeping, audit capabilities and overall standardisation of warfarin management in many clinics. However, training of the operator is still of paramount importance as human intervention at times will be needed and a balance must be struck between the operator not overruling all computer derived decisions but at the same time recognising the need to intervene, such as in circumstances of alcohol consumption, missed doses, changes in medication or doses of medication and starting/stopping medication.

Table 5h. Dose adjustments for upper therapeutic range INR 3.0 – 4.0 when over-anticoagulated

Over-anticoagulated		Dose Adjustment	Next Appointment
Slight	4.1- 4.3	Continue as before	As before, but max 4 weeks
Moderate	4.4 - 4.7	Omit dose for 1 day	2-4 weeks
Significant	4.8 - 5.3	Omit doses for 2 days	1-2 weeks
Severe	5.4 - 5.9	Omit doses for 2 days	1 week
Very severe	6.0 - 7.0	Omit warfarin for 3 days	Next day
	>7.0	Omit warfarin and administer Vit K Follow 'Management of Over Anticoagulation' guideline	Next day

Evidence of bleeding may require a change in this schedule, or referral to a Haematologist, at any INR

Interrupting Treatment for Surgery "Perioperative Bridging"

In recent years there has been increasing interest in Perioperative Bridging, the temporary interruption of warfarin therapy with short-term parenteral anticoagulants that have a rapid onset/offset especially for surgery or an invasive procedure to reduce the risk of thromboembolism. For surgery the risk of perioperative bleeding if warfarin is continued must be balanced against the risk of thromboembolism if warfarin is stopped [119].

There have been no randomised studies in this field and again local guidelines should try to reflect best clinical practice. Stratification of patients into different risk groups is essential and the guidelines should be as clear and simple as possible. Care should be taken in patients with mechanical heart valves as none of the low molecular weight heparins are licensed for this indication and often it is difficult to know if the valve is of the “older” or “newer” type. The original caged-ball valves are more thrombogenic than tilting disc valves, whilst the bileaflet valves are the least thrombogenic. In the absence of other factors requiring systemic anticoagulation, patients receiving autografts, homografts or bioprosthetic valves do not require long term anticoagulation but do require treatment with antiplatelet agents and 3-month oral anticoagulation after surgery [120]. For these reasons and to limit confusion all valve patients should be considered very high risk and given unfractionated heparin. An example of such a protocol from Guy’s and St Thomas’ NHS Foundation Trust is illustrated below in Figure 13.

Therapeutic Uses

Warfarin is prescribed for patients with an increased tendency for thrombosis or as secondary prophylaxis in individuals with documented thrombotic disease.

Deep Vein Thrombosis (DVT) and Pulmonary Embolism (PE)

Prevention: Low molecular weight heparins are the preferred drugs for the prevention of perioperative thrombosis as it is immediate acting with a short half-life, although randomised controlled trials validating this approach are lacking. However a limited use for warfarin may exist in situations where the risk of thrombosis is very high but its main role is in longer-term treatment.

Treatment: Oral anticoagulants prevent early thrombus extension and embolism and minimise late recurrence. Initially, unfractionated heparin is given and warfarin therapy added once the diagnosis is confirmed. The two drugs are overlapped for at least four days until the INR has exceeded 2.0 for two or more days [121] after which heparin can be discontinued.

Trials have found that initial treatment with a fixed dose of low molecular weight heparin is no less effective or less safe than standard unfractionated heparin therapy in the treatment of a DVT [122-125]. Data from Kuijer *et al* [122] are shown below in Table 6. This in turn has made home management of a DVT possible, which is preferred by many patients.

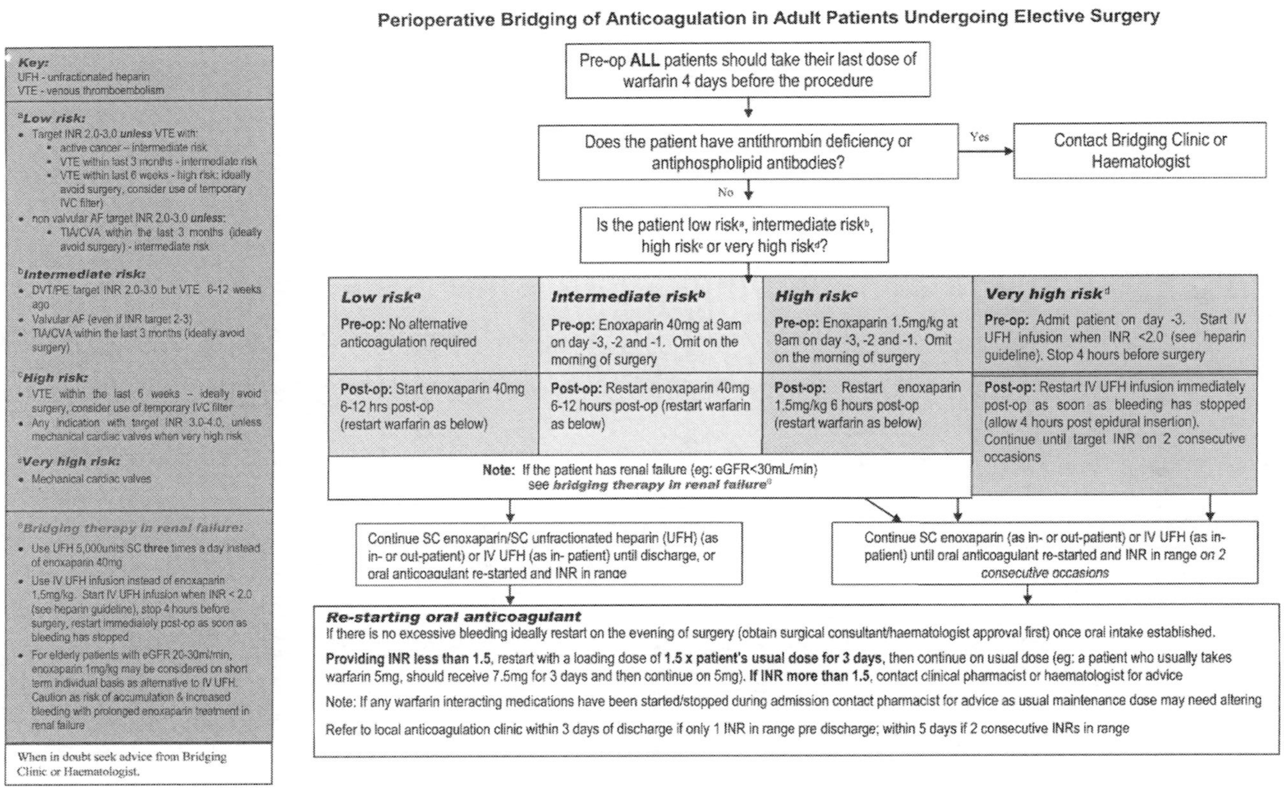

Figure 13. Example perioperative bridging protocol. Reproduced with permission from the Centre for Haemostasis & Thrombosis, Guy's & St. Thomas' NHS foundation Trust, London, UK.

At present the treatment of PE should be confined to a hospital setting at least for the first 48 hours. Treatment for pulmonary embolism is typically provided in a hospital, where the patients' condition can be closely monitored, as the clinical severity of a PE can be highly variable.

This can range from asymptomatic to severe hypoxemia, right ventricular failure, shock, and death. As a result, great clinical judgment is required and death from a pulmonary embolism is often fatal [126].

Table 6. LMWH vs UFH in the treatment of DVT

Preparation	Total number of patients (LMWH)	% cases with VTE (LMWH)	Total number of patients (UFH)	% cases with VTE (UFH)
Nadroparin (Fraxiparine®)	361	5.5	355	9.0
Tinzaparin (Innohep®)	213	2.8	219	6.9
Enoxaparin (Clexane®)	314	4.1	320	6.3
Dalteparin (Fragmin®)	322	5.0	339	2.4

Symptomatic recurrent venous thromboembolic complications during initial treatment and during 3-month to 6-month follow-up. Data taken from [122]. LMWH, low molecular weight heparin; UFH, unfractionated heparin; DVT, deep vein thrombosis; VTE, venous thromboembolism.

Established treatment with warfarin after a thrombosis is usually for 3 to 6 months but there is growing evidence that patients' clinical presentation should determine the optimal duration. Six to twelve weeks treatment is probably enough when a DVT follows surgery or transient immobilization, such as "a leg in a cast" or "a secondary or provoked" event, as a recurrence is minimal after six weeks of treatment for a symptomatic calf vein thrombosis and by three months for a proximal DVT [127].

In contrast, treatment for longer than six months may be required after an "idiopathic" or "unprovoked" DVT, recurrent thrombotic events, or when there is a continuing cause like cancer or an inherited or acquired thrombophilia [128,129]. Whether treatment should be given for one year, two years, or life long remains open to discussion but the bleeding risk should not be disregarded in this. Indeed the 8th ACCP guidelines do advocate life long anticoagulation after a first unprovoked event.

Problems Associated with the Management of DVT

When suspecting a deep vein thrombosis (DVT) of the lower extremity, a number of questions should be considered. These include:

- Consider the differential diagnosis and risk factors for a DVT?
- What is the best way to diagnose or exclude a thrombosis?
- Which initial therapy to use and is hospitalisation required?
- What is the duration of treatment (e.g. agent used, monitoring, INR range and length of time of anticoagulation)?
- Should one screen for a thrombophilia in the patient and family members?

Calf Vein Thrombosis

It is commonly believed that calf vein thromboses are clinically unimportant but the possibility of extension and embolism should not be forgotten. There is evidence to suggest that recurrence during a three month period after a proven calf vein thrombosis is up to 23% in those untreated as opposed to 0% in those treated [130]. Therefore a detected calf vein thrombosis should be treated unless there are contraindications.

Diagnostic Tests for DVT

Compression ultrasonography has now replaced venography as a first-line diagnostic test. This in conjunction with a scoring system and D-dimer analysis has lead to the establishment of guided flow charts for the diagnosis of DVTs.

The Wells scoring systems for DVT [131,132] and PE [133] are commonly employed, examples of which are presented in Tables 7 and 8 respectively and an example flow chart as Figure 14.

Other pretest probability scoring systems are available, including the Hamilton score [134] and the Primary Care Rule (AMUSE score) proposed for use in primary care patients [135], however the Wells score for DVT (ie, Wells criteria for DVT) is most commonly used.

Table 7. DVT pre-test probability score

Clinical feature	Score
Active malignancy (treatment is on-going, within previous 6 months or palliative)	1
Paralysis, paresis or recent plaster immobilisation of the lower extremeties	1
Recently confined to bed >3 days or major surgery within 4 weeks	1
Localized tenderness along the distribution of the deep venous system	1
Entire leg swollen	1
Calf swelling by >3 cm when compared to the asymptomatic leg (measured below tibial tuberosity)	1
Pitting oedema (greater in symptomatic leg)	1
Collateral superficial veins (non-varicose)	1
Previous DVT	1
Alternative diagnosis to DVT as likely or more likely	-2
Score	
DVT unlikely	≤1
DVT likely	≥2

DVT, deep vein thrombosis.

Table 8. PE pre-test probability score

Clinical feature	Score
Clinical signs and symptoms of DVT	3.0
Alternative diagnosis of PE is less likely	3.0
Heart rate >100 beats/min	1.5
Immobilisation in previous 4 weeks	1.5
Surgery in previous 4 weeks	1.5
Previous DVT/PE	1.5
Active malignancy (treatment is on-going, within previous 6 months or palliative)	1.0
Haemoptysis	1.0
Score	
Low probability of PE	<2.0
Moderate probability of PE	2.0–6.0
High probability of PE	>6.0

DVT, deep vein thrombosis; PE, pulmonary embolism.

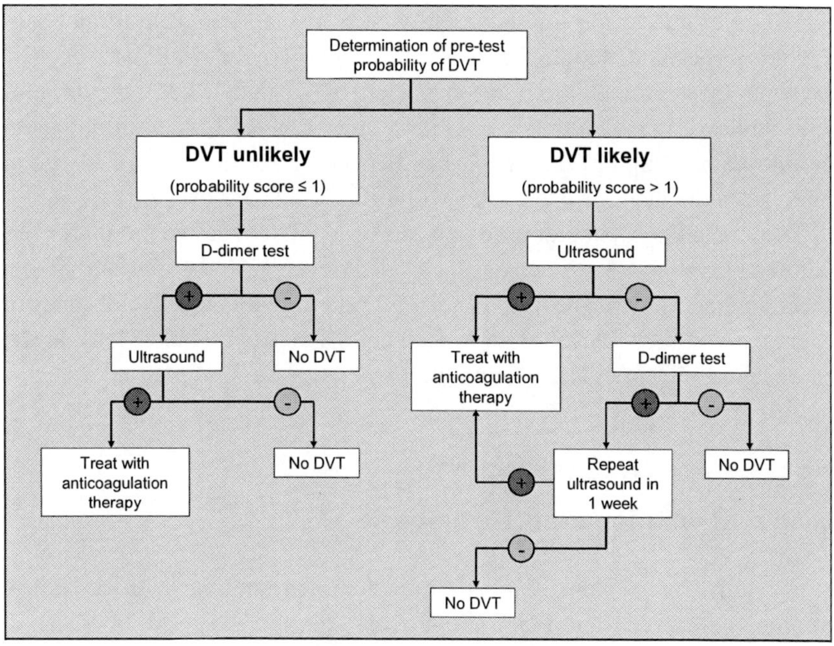

Figure 14. Diagnostic algorithm using D-dimer testing and ultrasound imaging in patients with suspected DVT. (DVT, deep vein thrombosis).

Table 9. Conditions other than DVT/PE that can lead to D-dimer elevation

Recent surgery
Disseminated intravascular coagulation
Acute myocardial infarction
Unstable angina
Atrial fibrillation
Acute aortic dissection
Vasculitis
Acute cerebrovascular accident
Infection/sepsis
Malignancy (i.e. lung, prostate, cervical, colorectal)
Concurrent systemic illness
Vaso-occlusive sickle cell crisis
Superficial phlebitis
Pregnancy
Age >60 years

However due to the limited sensitivity to a small calf vein thrombosis, a negative ultrasound should be repeated once or twice within a seven day period in case there is proximal extension of an undetected calf thrombus. With duplex ultrasonography, the detection of a calf vein thrombosis is possible with a single scan and hence depending on the type of ultra-sonography used the diagnostic pathway will differ.

D-dimer analysis is best used in terms of its high negative predictive value with respect to DVT/PE because elevated levels can be present in other conditions, as shown above in Table 9. Additionally, small clots may not generate a sufficient elevation to exceed cut-off values and clots >10 days old can reach a physiological equilibrium whereby the D-dimer levels appear normal.

Recurrent or Idiopathic Thrombosis

A study by Schulman *et al* in patients presenting with a recurrent thrombosis showed that indefinite therapy (target INR 2.0 to 2.85) was associated with a significantly lower incidence of recurrent disease at four years (2.6 versus 20.7 percent in those treated for six months, relative risk 0.13, 95% CI 0.04-0.40) and a trend to a higher risk for major haemorrhage (8.6 versus 2.7 percent; relative risk 3.3 95% CI 0.9-10) [128]. However, ongoing treatment increased the rate of major bleeding during this period from 2.7% to 8.6%, while mortality remained unchanged. The patient should also be informed of the estimated incidence of major bleeding should warfarin be continued. In a large meta-analysis, the rate of major bleeding if anticoagulation was continued beyond three months was 2.7 per 100 patient-years, with a case fatality rate of 9.1 percent (95% CI 2.5-22) [137].

In a separate study by Kearon *et al* comparing three months to a longer period of treatment after a first "idiopathic" thrombosis, there was recurrence in 16 of 77 patients during ten months of follow-up, compared with only 1 of 76 patients respectively [138]. However, the annual risk of major bleeding was increased from zero to 4%. Hence the high risk of bleeding necessitates the need for careful risk assessment when considering a patient for long term treatment. Patients who experience a second thrombotic event when on warfarin and who were in the therapeutic range at this time need long term anticoagulation within an INR range of 3.0 to 4.0.

Atrial Fibrillation

The use of warfarin in healthy patients to prevent systemic embolism with atrial fibrillation (AF) is now widely used and increasing. From clinical trials the annual risk of a first ischaemic stroke is reduced by almost 70% (from 7% to 3% per annum) Mortality is reduced by 33% with a small increase in serious bleeding (from 1.0% to 1.3% per annum) [139,140].

The prevalence of AF rises from about 3% at age 65 to more than 10% by age 85 and a very important determinant of ischaemic stroke in AF patients is age [140]. In a cross-sectional study of almost 1.9 million men and women, the prevalence of atrial fibrillation was shown to increase with age, ranging from 0.1 for those less than 55 years of age to over 9 percent in those ≥85 years of age [141]. At all ages, the prevalence was higher in men than women (Table 10).

Table 10. Prevalence of atrial fibrillation stratified by age and gender

Age range (y)	Women % with AF (n)		Men % with AF (n)	
<55	*0.1*	(530)	*0.2*	(1259)
55 – 59	*0.4*	(310)	*0.9*	(634)
60 – 64	*1.0*	(566)	*1.7*	(934)
65 – 69	*1.7*	(896)	*3.0*	(1426)
70 – 74	*3.4*	(1498)	*5.0*	(1907)
75 – 79	*5.0*	(1572)	*7.3*	(1886)
80 – 84	*7.2*	(1291)	*10.3*	(1374)
≥85	*9.1*	(1132)	*11.1*	(759)

Data from [141]

A study by Wolf *et al* showed that AF accounts for about 1.5% of all strokes in patients aged 50-59 years, and almost 25% of strokes in patients aged 80 - 89 years [142]. Other risk factors including previous stroke, transient ischaemic attack, diabetes, treated hypertension, heart failure, ischaemic heart disease, left atrium hypertrophy and left ventricular dysfunction should also be assessed [143].

The risk of stroke accumulates with these additional risk factors and hence a young patient with none of these and isolated AF should be considered low risk with their annual risk of stroke being <1%. A study by Frost *et al* [143] showed that the rate of subsequent stroke (percent per patient per year) was:

- 1.3 in those aged 50 to 59 years
- 2.2 in those aged 60 to 69 years
- 4.2 for those aged 70 to 79 years
- 5.1 for those aged 80 to 89 years

Each AF patient should have the relative risk assessed for stroke versus bleeding when long term anticoagulation is being considered and the best target INR determined. With an INR of <2.0 the risk of bleeding is reduced but that of stroke increases.

Below 2.0, the relative risk doubles at 1.7, becomes three times at 1.5, six times at 1.3, and reaches eighteen times at a normal INR. However there is no gain beyond an INR of 2.0 [144] and some benefits are to found with an INR of 1.5 to 1.9. This target range may be appropriate for those patients aged above 75 who run with a high INR both of which increase the risk of intracranial or major bleeding.

The $CHADS_2$ score is a clinical prediction rule used for determining the need for anticoagulant therapy, and if so, which type, by estimating the risk of stroke in patients with non-rheumatic AF [145]. Adding together the points that correspond to specific conditions that a patient has generates the $CHADS_2$ score. Table 11 below details the scoring system and Table 12 the risk levels and anticoagulation considerations.

The CHA_2DS_2-VASc score extends the $CHADS_2$ score by including the additional common stroke risk factors listed below, each attracting one point [146].

- age 65-74
- female gender
- vascular disease.

Table 11. $CHADS_2$ score for atrial fibrillation stroke risk

C	Congestive heart failure (recent)	+1
H	Hypertension	+1
A	Age $\geq$ 75 yrs	+1
D	Diabetes mellitus	+1
S_2	Stroke or transient ischaemic attacks (TIA) previously	+2

Table 12. $CHADS_2$ scores, stroke risk, risk levels and anticoagulation considerations

$CHADS_2$ score	Stroke risk per 100 pt-yr	$CHADS_2$ risk level	Warfarin recommended	Anticoagulation considerations
0	1.9	Low	No	Aspirin daily
1	2.8	Low	No	
2	4.0	Moderate	Yes	Warfarin with target range INR 2.0-3.0 unless contraindicated (e.g. clinically significant GI bleeding, inability to obtain regular INR screening)
3	5.9	Moderate	Yes	
4	8.5	High	Yes	
5	12.5	High	Yes	
6	18.2	High	Yes	

In the CHA_2DS_2-VASc score, age ≥ 75 yrs is accorded an extra weighting of 2 points. Thus, the maximum CHA_2DS_2-VASc score is 9 compared to 6 for $CHADS_2$. Patients with a CHA_2DS_2-VASc score of zero are truly a low risk and the recommendation is not to prescribe antithrombotic therapy, or at most, aspirin at 75-325mg daily. A score of 1 is considered moderate risk and warfarin with a target INR range of 2.0 – 3.0, new oral anticoagulant (i.e. dabigatran) or aspirin at 75-325mg daily are recommended. A score of ≥2 is considered high risk and warfarin with a target INR range of 2.0 – 3.0 or new oral anticoagulant are recommended. The 70% risk reduction in stroke with warfarin is far superior to that of aspirin alone at 30% and aspirin should perhaps be reserved for those uncomplicated AF patients with a low baseline risk of embolism. In patients where the bleeding risk is high, aspirin although less effective than warfarin might be safer.

Cardio-Embolic Stroke Prevention in Conditions Other Than AF

At least 4 weeks of anticoagulation should be given to cardiac arrhythmia patients prior to cardio-version to minimise systemic embolism [140]. After myocardial infarction (MI) three to six months of anticoagulation should be given if intra-ventricular thrombus is present or to prevent this if other risk factors are present, which include transmural anterior infarcts or left ventricular dysfunction. Indeed there may be a good case for long term anticoagulation in ongoing left ventricular dysfunction. Small observational studies have suggested a reduction in the stroke rate in patients treated with warfarin [147]. However the evidence in severe left ventricular dysfunction to support the sole use of warfarin or aspirin is limited and should be interpreted with caution, as concluded in two systematic reviews by the Cochrane database [147,148].

Prosthetic Heart Valves

Systemic embolism remains the main source of mortality and morbidity in prosthetic mechanical heart valves and life long anticoagulation is still recommended despite the fact that improved design and materials have greatly reduced their thrombogenicity. The type of valve, its position and whether both mitral and aortic valves have been replaced influence the risk, which is higher with mitral valves. By contrast tissue valves, with the exception of the first three months, are almost free of thromboembolic complications [149]. In general and assuming there are no contraindications, the older and more thrombogenic models (caged ball or disc) should be considered very high risk and kept in the higher INR target range of 3.0 to 4.0. Newer valves with a lower risk (bileaflet or tilting disc) can be kept in the range 2.0 to 3.0.

By the addition of aspirin the risk of systemic embolism can be further reduced. However with a 2.5 times increase in major gastrointestinal bleeding [150] the use of this combination should probably only be considered in patients who are at a very high risk of systemic thromboembolism, which would include those with more than one mechanical valve, previous embolism or associated AF [149].

Special Circumstances for Anticoagulation - Antiphospholipid Antibody Syndrome

This cohort of patients often requires specialist input as both the management of their anticoagulation and the primary condition can be complex and difficult to control. For this reason it is extremely difficult to make a firm recommendation about the optimal target range for this condition. Some studies have suggested that the prevention of venous and/or arterial thrombosis in this group is only achievable if the INR is kept above 3.0 whereas others has maintained that a lower INR is successful in this. Depending on the individual circumstances of the patient the INR range should be tailored on an individual basis. The role of aspirin in preventing thrombosis in antiphospholipid syndrome is unclear.

MODELS FOR MANAGING ANTICOAGULATION

Over the years as the number of patients requiring anticoagulation has increased, different models and approaches to running anticoagulation clinics and managing patients have evolved. When used appropriately treatment with oral anticoagulants has been shown to potentially save lives, reduce patient harm and at the same time reduce overall healthcare costs [151]. However, long term management plans maximising the benefits and reducing the risks are influenced greatly by the method of management which plays a vital role in safety and efficacy of treatment. Throughout this evolution these different approaches have had both positive and negative qualities and indeed today different combinations of these may be used. Good anticoagulation control results in improved outcomes, with a decrease in the incidence of bleeding and thromboembolic events. The outcome of oral anticoagulation therapy (OAT) is dependent on the model of care used to manage warfarin treatment and better outcomes are associated with the use of a specialised anticoagulation management service (AMS), computerised decision support and increased testing frequency, which can be facilitated by patient self-testing (PST) of the INR. The goal of this is to achieve Systematic Anticoagulation Management (SAM), which is POCT by a healthcare provider in a clinic or GP surgery or by the patient. This approach involves the patient's participation with physicians in their own anticoagulation management and is a patient-focused approach to anticoagulation management that utilises PT/INR testing at the point of care. This POCT can involve a conventional laboratory or a point-of-care device. However care should be taken when employing a combination of both as the INR results will vary between each method. The components of a SAM include:

1. Direct, active management – one healthcare professional to coordinate patient care and provide continuing patient education and quality control
2. Patient scheduling and tracking: an integrated system to schedule patient testing, track results, and flag missed appointments
3. Accessible, accurate, frequent PT/INR testing; may increase a patients' time in the therapeutic range (TTR); POCT devices allow for

instant PT/INR ratio results to facilitate implementation of effective management models

4. Patient-specific decision support and interaction; focuses on individual patient care and provides continuing communication regarding therapy

The days of a single handed practitioner seeing sixty to eighty patients in a morning with hand written paper records and an empirical approach to dosing together with a Biomedical Scientist performing manual PT measurements in a water bath is not so long ago. The introduction of portable POCT devices in the 1980s provided an alternative approach for the management of anticoagulation treatment.

Approaches to Anticoagulation Management

A variety of models exist for managing patients on oral anticoagulants, which can essentially be divided into the following categories, all of which can employ POCT or conventional testing methods or a combination thereof.

Hospital Based Anticoagulation Clinics

Keeping patients on oral anticoagulants within a narrow therapeutic range requires expert dose management. Because of the intensity of the management required, anticoagulation clinics were developed to help physicians manage these patients, keeping a focus on the narrow therapeutic range required to minimise adverse events.

These centralised specialty clinics with particular expertise in anti-coagulation have demonstrated improvements in quality of care, improved patient compliance and reduced complications compared with routine management. However they are often very busy and necessitate the patient traveling to a hospital clinic.

Different models can exist in this from traditional "face to face" clinics with the patient waiting to be seen or a "postal" service where the patient is bled but then goes and any communication is done by telephone and the record book posted back to the patient.

Ambulatory Based Anticoagulation Clinics

Increasingly GPs, local Pharmacists and now Polyclinics are becoming involved in the treatment and management of anticoagulation therapy. Patient testing can be performed by a conventional laboratory and results are interpreted and managed entirely by his or her own GP. However, ambulatory services generally only want stable uncomplicated patients, which of course, depending on circumstances can become unstable and hence returned to the hospital setting.

Patient Self Monitoring and Management

The approval of several POCT devices for home use has extended the potential to further improve patient outcomes. These devices allow for more frequent monitoring to assess time in therapeutic range and to detect any drift in INR prior to a clinically significant event. Patients are actively involved in their own care, which may lead to a better understanding of how lifestyle can impact INR stability. In addition, the consistency of instrumentation and reagents may provide more reliable INR measurements that usual care or a systematic care model cannot achieve [152]. Patients can monitor their own INR at home and receive dose adjustments from their physician, or after proper training, adjust their own dose [153]. Data suggest that patients achieve significantly better outcomes than those receiving usual care from their physicians but only slightly better outcomes than focused care delivered by an anticoagulation clinic [153,154]. Patient selection and training is an important component of successful self-testing [154-156]. There are barriers to self-testing. In a national survey of anticoagulation practitioners in the USA almost 60% of anticoagulation clinics had policies and procedures prohibiting patient self-testing [157]. Fewer than 1% of the patients managed by these anticoagulation clinics used self-testing. The primary barriers were cost of the device (78.7%), cost of reagent cartridges (60.4%) and fear that self-testing might lead to unintended self-management (35.7%).

The majority of the existing trials have various methodological problems. Heneghan *et al* reviewed 14 randomised, controlled clinical trials with measured endpoints of major hemorrhage, thromboembolic events, death, tests in range, minor hemorrhage, test frequency and feasibility of self-monitoring [158]. Each of the trials alone was not statistically significant, but combining them showed that you get a benefit in terms of mortality [158]. However, self-management of oral anticoagulant therapy appeared at least as good as, and possibly better than conventional management in "highly" selected patients.

OPTIMISING MANAGEMENT STRATEGIES

None of these management models inherently provide systematic active management of anticoagulation therapy. It is the combination of an active management system with the structural model of management appropriate for the individual patient that will result in optimal anticoagulation management. Although each has merits a potential problem with these functioning in isolation is a lack of communication and hence information as they may be using different computer systems, POCT methods and have non-standardised guidelines. For the optimised delivery of anticoagulation therapy, the following 9 key areas have been identified irrespective of the structure and setting in which the care is delivered [159]:

- Qualifications of personnel
- Supervision
- Care management and coordination
- Documentation
- Patient education
- Patient selection and assessment
- Laboratory monitoring
- Initiation and stabilisation of warfarin therapy
- Maintenance of therapy

Systematic anticoagulation management has been shown to reduce thromboembolic and hemorrhagic events, improving patient outcomes and reducing associated healthcare costs [152,160] Further to this patient satisfaction is high and the opportunity to provide more efficient patient care with reduced labour-related costs is significant [161]. If not managed well, treatment with oral anticoagulants is associated with a high complication rate and good management requires keeping the patient in a narrow therapeutic INR range. Focused anticoagulation clinic management has been shown to improve outcomes compared to the routine management provided by physicians. A combination of these models could possibly be more beneficial and would fit with current day thinking on ambulatory services and patient participation and choice. A collaborative network might be possible between the hospital clinic, ambulatory services and the patient, which for simplicity could be visualised as a "Hub and Spoke" The traditional hospital anti-coagulation clinic taking on a "Hub" status with responsibility for centralising record keeping, maintaining working guidelines and training and education of both patients and practitioners. Figure 15 depicts an integrated approach of these service models.

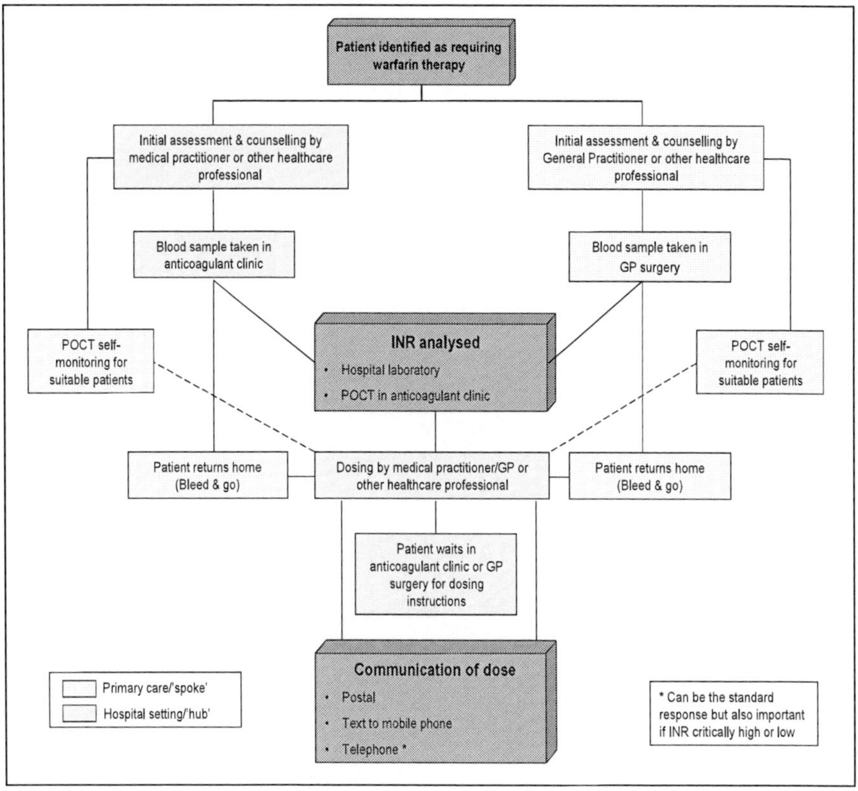

Figure 15. Integrated warfarin monitoring. Patients can be assessed and stabilised in the hospital setting and either continue to be monitored there or can choose to be monitored in a primary care setting with support from the hospital as appropriate. Suitable patients can self-monitor with point of care testing (POCT), some even becoming trained to self-adjust their dose when INR results are within a defined range and only contacting healthcare professionals if outside range.

The responsibility for in-patient anticoagulation services could then also be undertaken. The "Spoke" then provides ease of accessibility with standardised treatment across the network. Central to this is the necessity to have a robust networked IT system.

Chapter 5

BEYOND STANDARD MONITORING

DETERMINANTS OF THERAPEUTIC WARFARIN DOSING

An interplay of many factors determines an individual's therapeutic warfarin dose requirement. When 4-hydroxycoumarin drugs were first used clinically, very few of these factors had been identified. In 1959 Karl Link listed factors that he thought important [4]. Those that were proved correct are listed below:

a) The vitamin K levels in the diet affect not only the intensity but also the duration of the anticoagulant action
b) Nutritional status affects anticoagulant response – fasting generally enhances the effect (likely to be connected with point i)
c) The use of salicylates (aspirin) augmented the response
d) Hepatic and renal function influences both the intensity and duration of the response
e) The presence of drugs that affect the total functioning capacity of the liver e.g. theophyllin and digitalis
f) Pregnant or lactating females show a slight resistance to the drug's anticoagulant action.

Patients with a very high warfarin requirement, and conversely patients with extreme sensitivity to warfarin were identified, and first described by O'Reilly and Bays in 1964 and 1965 respectively [162,163]. This broad spectrum of responsiveness could not be fully explained by Link's preliminary list of determinants, and many further factors have been identified in the past half century, as depicted in Figure 16 below.

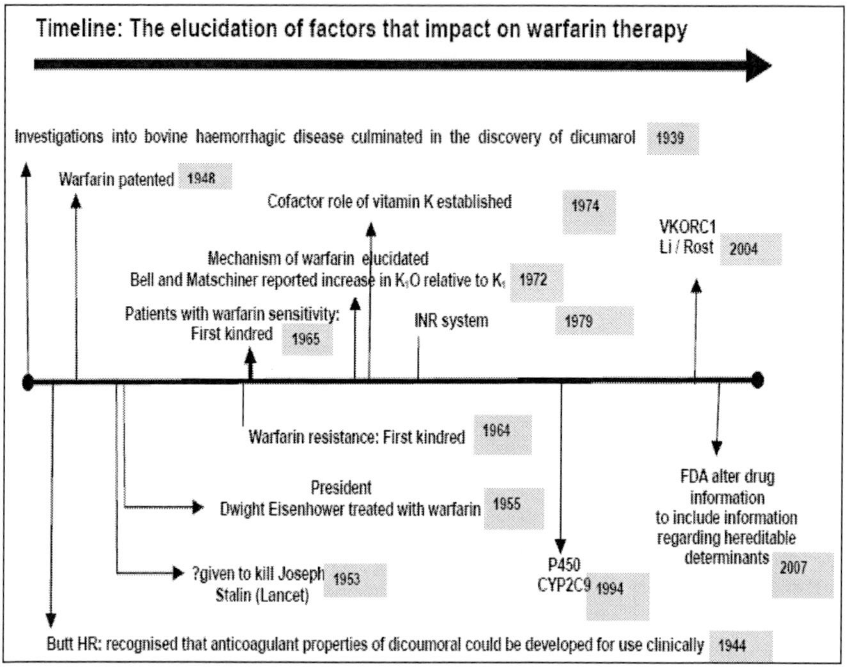

Figure 16. Timeline of discoveries of factors impacting on warfarin therapy.

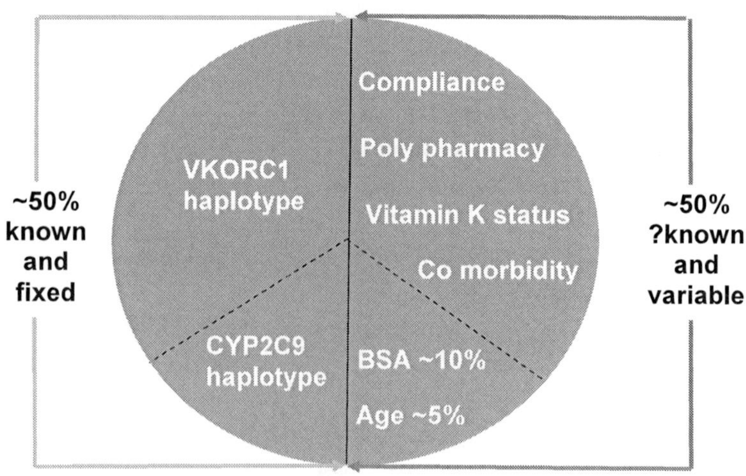

Figure 17. Determinants of warfarin dose requirement. BSA, body surface area.

Some determinants of warfarin dose requirement are fixed e.g. genotype, and their impact is well characterised. Other factors change in a predicable fashion e.g. the impact of a patient's age. Other factors can have a transient effect making safe and therapeutic anticoagulation difficult, as depicted above in Figure 17.

Molecular Determinants of Warfarin Dose Requirement

Molecular determinants with the largest impact on warfarin dose requirement are cytochrome P-450 2C9 isoenzyme (CYP2C9) and vitamin K epoxide reductase subunit 1 (VKORC1). More than 30 genes have been reported as possibly having an impact on warfarin dosing. Other notable molecular determinants include nucleotide substitutions in the genes that encode Factors II, VII and IX, γ-Carboxylase and apolipoprotein E (Apo E).

Cytochrome P-450 2C9 Isoenzyme

The cytochrome P-450 2C9 isoenzyme (CYP2C9) is a 60-kDa liver microsomal protein that has a major role in the oxidation of both xenobiotic and endogenous compounds and makes up about 18% of the cytochrome P450 cytochrome protein [164]. The gene that encodes CYP2C9 has been mapped to chromosome 10 (q24.2) and contains 9 exons. Warfarin is used clinically as a racemic mixture of S and R enantiomers, with the S-enantiomer accounting for the majority of the therapeutic effect (x3-5 *vs.* R-). Several cytochrome P-450 isoenzymes (CYP1A2, CYP3A4, CYP2C19 and carbonyl reductase) catabolise R-warfarin. S-warfarin is predominantly catabolised by CYP2C9 generating 7-hydroxy and 6-hydroxy metabolites that lack any anticoagulant effect, and are quickly excreted in the urine.

CYP2C9 is highly polymorphic with more than 50 variants described in ethnic populations. In Caucasians, common CYP2C9 haplotypes include CYP2C9*2 (c.C416T, p.Arg144Cys exon3; allele frequency 12%) and *3 (c.A1061C, p.Ile359Leu, exon 7; allele frequency 8%). Both these variants confer diminished clearance of S-warfarin leading to over anticoagulation when doses of warfarin more appropriate for the reference sequence (wild type allele) CYP2C9*1 homozygotes are used. Percentage dose reductions relative to CYP2C9 genotype are shown in Figure 18. This mode of action can therefore be classified as pharmacokinetic. It is thought that CYP2C9 genotype accounts for approximately 15% of a patient's warfarin dose requirement.

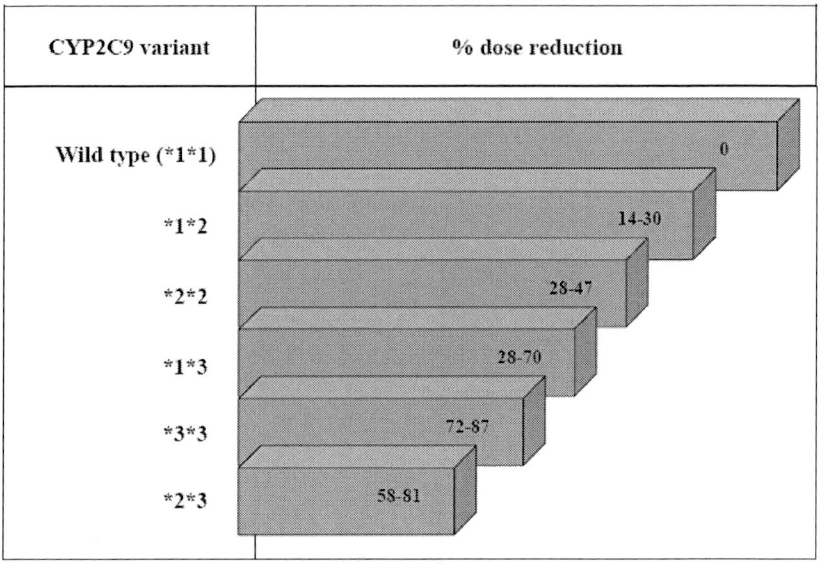

Figure 18. Warfarin dose reduction and CYP2C9 genotype.

Patients with warfarin sensitivity as a consequence of their CYP2C9 genotype can be successfully managed with lower doses of warfarin but do take longer to achieve stable and therapeutic anticoagulation. They require move intensive monitoring, partly because algorithms applied to the care of these patients have been tailored for patients with a more standard response. These patients are more likely to have a bleeding episode in the first few months of anticoagulation and also more likely to suffer a thrombotic event.

VKORC1

The gene that encodes the enzymatically active component of the VKOR complex has been identified on chromosome 16 (16p12-q21). VKORC1 is the molecular target of coumarin anticoagulants. The expressed enzyme is 163 amino acids long with at least three transmembrane domains within the endoplasmic reticulum. A shorter variant (isoform 2) which is 156 amino acids long has also been identified. Polymorphisms within this gene are a major pharmacodynamic determinant of warfarin dose response and it is estimated that VKORC1 genotype accounts for up to 40% of a patient's warfarin dose requirement. Bioinformatic [165] and site-directed mutagenesis [166] investigations have pointed to cysteine residues 132 and 135 in TM3 as the probable redox centre in VKORC1 responsible for the salvaging of K_1O to K_1 and a TYA motif at residues 138–140 also in TM3, as the main coumarin binding site [167].

Individuals homozygous for the VKORC1 *2 haplotype have a lower warfarin dose requirement as a consequence of decreased hepatic expression of VKORC1 when compared with haplotypes VKORC1 *1, *3 or *4. Rare mutations have also been identified in patients with very high warfarin dose requirements (see warfarin resistance p 82-87). There is no evidence that VKORC1 mutations perturb vitamin K metabolism [168].

Other molecular determinants with a pharmacodynamic impact on warfarin dose requirement have been identified. The nucleotide substitution Thr165Met in the gene that encodes Factor II has been associated with an increased warfarin dose requirement as has the G-401T substitution in the gene that encodes Factor VII [169]. Nucleotide substitutions (Ala-10 → Thr) and (Ala → Val) in Factor IX confer a reduction in affinity of the carboxylase for the mutant propeptide. Affected patients have normal coagulation until challenged with warfarin. Once challenged with warfarin the patient's coagulation mimics symptoms of haemophilia B [170]. Inheritance of this disorder is X-chromosomal linked and although rare its prevalence is higher in certain populations e.g. those of Swiss German decent [171].

Other single nucleotide polymorphisms that may have a minor impact on warfarin dose requirement include those within the gene encoding γ-Carboxylase [172] and ApoE [173].

Environmental Determinants of Warfarin Dose

Vitamin K

Compounds with vitamin K activity have a common 2-methyl-1, 4-naphthoquinone nucleus and a variable alkyl substituent at the 3 position. The major naturally occurring K vitamins are the plant form phylloquinone (vitamin K_1) and multiple forms of menaquinones (vitamins K_2) of bacterial origin. K_1 has a 20-carbon, phytyl side chain whereas menaquinones have multi-prenyl side chains, their number being indicated by a suffix (i.e. menaquinone-n, abbreviated MK-n)

Sources of Vitamin K

In a typical Western diet, K_1 and multiple forms of menaquinones (vitamins K_2) of bacterial origin account for about 90% and 10% of vitamin K intakes respectively [172]. Dietary menaquinones mainly comprise of MK-4, MK-7, MK-8, and MK-9 [175], although menaquinones with longer side chains up to MK-13 are present in human liver [176,177].

Approximately 2000 foods have been assigned a provisional K_1 content [178,179]. An excerpt from the provisional UK data-base for K_1 content is shown below in Table 13.

Table 13. K_1 Content (μg/100g) of Common Foods

Concentration Ranges			
0.1-1.0	**1-10**	**10-100**	**100-1000**
Avocado (1.0)	Apples (6)	Beans, runner (26)	Broccoli tops (179)
Bananas (0.1)	Aubergines (6)	Beans, French (39)	Brussels sprouts (147)
Beef, steak (0.8)	Baked beans (3)	Beans, broad (19)	Cabbage, green (339)
Bread, white (0.4)	Barley (7)	Cabbage (19)	Kale (618)
Chicken, thigh (0.1)	Beef, corned (7)	Cauliflower (31)	Lettuce (129)
Coconut oil (0.5)	Beef, minced (2)	Chick peas (21)	Parsley (548)
Cod, fresh, fillet <0.1)	Bilberries (4)	Cucumber (21)	Rapeseed oil (123)
Cornflakes (<0.1)	Bran, wheat (10)	Greengages (15)	Soybean (173)
Flour, white (0.8)	Bread, wholemeal (2)	Mustard greens (Cress) (88)	Spinach (380)
Grapefruit (<0.1)	Butter (7)	Olive oil, extra virgin (80)	Watercress (315)
Ham, tinned (0.1)	Carrots (6)	Peas (34)	
Maize (0.3)	Cheese, various (2-6)		
Mangoes (0.5)	Chocolate, plain (2)		

Concentration Ranges			
0.1-1.0	**1-10**	**10-100**	**100-1000**
Melon, yellow (0.1)	Corn oil (3)		
Melon, water (0.3)	Courgettes (3)		
Milk, cows (0.6)	Cranberries (2)		
Mushrooms (0.3)	Cream, double (6)		
Oranges (<0.1)	Dates, fresh (6)		
Parsnips (<0.1)	Egg, yolk (2)		
Peanuts, roast (0.4)	Figs, fresh (3)		
Pilchards, brine (0.6)	Grapes, black (8)		
Pinapple (0.2)	Grapes, green (9)		
Pork, chop, lean (<0.1)	Leeks (10)		
Potatoes (0.9)	Liver, lamb (7)		
Rice, white (0.1)	Liver, ox (4)		
Rice, brown (0.8)	Nectarines (3)		
Salmon, tin, brine (0.1)	Oats (10)		
Sausage pork/beef (0.2)	Palm oil (8)		
Spaghetti (0.2)	Peaches, fresh (4)		
Tuna, tin, brine (0.3)	Pea (6)		
Turnips (0.2)	Peppers, green (6)		
Yoghurt (0.8)	Peppers, red (2)		
	Plums, red (8)		
	Raisins (4)		
	Rhubarb (4)		
	Safflower oil (3)		
	Strawberries (3)		
	Sunflower oil (6)		
	Swede (2)		
	Sunflower oil (6)		
	Swede (2)		
	Tomatoes (6)		
	Wheat (8)		

Data are for raw foods except were cooked form is indicated. Data taken from [179,180].

Dark-green leaved vegetables such as kale, parsley, spinach, cabbage, broccoli, Brussels sprouts and lettuce contribute the greatest proportion of daily vitamin K_1 intake [180,181]. Table 14 below shows percentage dietary intake of K_1 by main food groups from a study in a population from Dundee, Scotland. Other rich sources of this vitamin include some plant oils (e.g. rapeseed and olive oil), although K_1 is quickly lost if the oil is exposed to fluorescent light or sunlight.

Table 14. Dietary intakes (%) of K_1 by main food groups

	All	Men	Women
Cereals	14.3	15.1	13.7
Milks	3.7	4.3	3.3
Eggs	0.3	0.4	0.2
Vegetables	47.8	46.1	49.2
Meats	6.7	9.1**	4.5
Fruits	4.4	3.1	5.6*
Herbs/spices	0.7	0.8	0.6
Fish	2.3	2.1	2.5
Confectionary	1.0	1.0	0.9
Beverages	2.4	2.6	2.1
Misc.	10.9	9.7	12.0
Fats/Oils	5.4	5.6	5.2

Dietary intakes (%) of K_1 in a population from Dundee, Scotland by main food groups and sex (MAFF "Composition of Foods").* significant difference ($P < 0.05$), ** significant difference ($P < 0.01$) [181].

Much less information is available regarding the menaquinone content of foods. Dietary sources of menaquinones include animal meat, known to contain significant amounts of MK-4, and liver a source of long-chained menaquinones (100-200 μg/kg). Fermented food products such as cheese and curd cheese are rich sources (~50-200 μg/kg) of menaquinone-7, menaquinone-8 and menaquinone-9 [175], and Natto, a traditional Japanese food consisting of fermented bean curds, is a rich source of menaquinone-7 (10 mg/kg) [182].

Dietary Vitamin K Intakes in Oral nticoagulant Patients

Dietary intakes of vitamin K in patients on oral anticoagulant therapy are highly variable and often low [183]. Fluctuations in dietary vitamin K intake prevent stable anticoagulation with warfarin, with extremes of status having a clinical impact: pseudo resistance resulting from high dietary intakes; poor stability and increased sensitivity from low intakes. Attempts to improve anticoagulation control through the avoidance of vitamin K-rich foods may therefore inadvertently lead to poor control and compromise the status of other nutrients [183]. It has been suggested that daily supplements of vitamin K will decrease the impact of dietary variation and improve stability. Although two randomised, controlled trials have demonstrated that daily supplementation with 100 or 150 μg K1 improves anticoagulant stability, further larger trials are needed [184,185]. Others have considered whether the use of MK-7 a form of vitamin K made by bacteria may be better suited to this application since it may have more favourable kinetics [186].

MICROFLORAL SYNTHESIS OF MENAQUINONES

Microflora within the intestine produce considerable amounts of menaquinones and quantitative measurements of their concentrations at different sites have been made [187]. The production of menaquinones and other related isopreniod quinones, including demethylmenaquinones and ubiquinones has been reported in many different bacterial species, both anaerobic and aerobic, with each species producing distinct MK profiles [187]. The majority of MKs are found in the distal colon, with MK-10 the most abundant. However, it is difficult to envisage how in the absence of bile salts for solubilisation and absorption these highly lipophilic and bacterial membrane bound compounds can contribute to human vitamin K status [176]. A survey of 90 organisms found commonly in the human intestinal tract identified *E. Coli, B. Fragilis,* and *Eubacteria* as major producers of MKs [188]. In the rat, long chain MKs are utilised through coprophagy, (ingestion of faecal matter), and subsequent second passage through the bowel and concomitant absorption in the upper region of the small bowel [189]. There is some evidence in humans that colonic MK-4 is absorbed via the portal pathway [180], but the abundance of MKs in the human liver e.g. MK-10-13 remains unexplained. The likelihood that these originate from the intestine is increased by their absence from commonly eaten foods and that the MK producing anaerobic genus *Bacteroides*, which produces MK-10 and MK-11, are major inhabitants of the intestinal tract. The terminal ileum and caecum also contain MKs, produced by intestinal bacteria. The MKs present in this part of the gastro-intestinal tract could explain the presence of long-chain menaquinones in the liver, and may contribute to vitamin K status [187]. The menquinone content of post mortem human liver (mean ng/g ± SEM, wet weight) from individuals whom prior to death were receiving a broad spectrum of antibiotics for at least 5 days was significantly lower than individuals who were not taking antibiotics (214 ±

140 ng/g vs. 470 ± 150 ng/g respectively), suggesting that ingestion of antibiotics had altered the gut microflora and the subsequent absorption of the MKs [187]. Further evidence for the role of MKs derived from the intestinal tract in maintaining coagulation homeostasis has been gained from several studies showing that starvation or ingestion of vitamin K deficient diets does not readily induce vitamin K deficiency (as defined by changes in prothrombin time or clotting factor assays). Frick found that starvation of a group of patients who had suffered cerebral apoplexy over a period of 4-5 weeks did not induce vitamin K deficiency, while starvation combined with antibiotic therapy induced significant deficiency in 3-4 weeks [190].

POLY PHARMACY

More than 130 drug interactions with warfarin have so far been described [191]. The most common mechanism through which therapeutic anticoagulation is disturbed is the induction of the cytochrome P-450 2C9 isoenzyme by drugs that share common catabolic pathways with warfarin e.g. the antiepileptic drugs phenytoin and carbamazepine. This leads to an accelerated clearance of warfarin and a reduced anticoagulant effect. Conversely, the anti-arrhythmic agent amiodarone increases the anticoagulant effect of warfarin through the inhibition of P450 2C9.

Several cephalosporins, a class of β-lactam antibiotics originally derived from *Acremonium*, are associated with hypoprothrombinemia. Examples include latamoxef, cefmenoxime, moxalactam, cefoperazone, cefamandole, cefmetazole, and cefotetan. This is thought to be because of the N-methylthiotetrazole (NMTT) side chain of these cephalosporins, which blocks the enzyme vitamin K epoxide reductase [192].

It is not only prescription-type medications that have the capacity to prevent stable and therapeutic anticoagulation. The antiplatelet effect of aspirin increases the risk of bleeding when combined with warfarin. As a consequence of the risks associated with the combined use of aspirin with warfarin, Paracetamol (acetaminophen) is in the main considered to be the analgesic of choice for patients undergoing oral anticoagulant therapy. However, interactions have been reported with therapeutic doses of paracetamol after prolonged use of several days. Prolonged intake leads to an accumulation of N-acetyl-para-benzoquinoneimine (NAPQ1), the hepatotoxic metabolite. NAPQI interferes with the enzymes that drive the vitamin K cycle – in particular gamma-carboxylase [193].

Bulk-forming laxatives reduce the absorption of warfarin, whilst stimulant laxatives may decrease vitamin K absorption leading to an increase in the anticoagulation effect. Complementary healthcare products containing St John's Wort diminish warfarin action by increasing the elimination rate through induction of cytochrome P450 isoenzymes in the liver and gut (predominately CYP 3A4, but 1A2 and 2C9 activity also increased). Drinking large quantities of cranberry juice has also been linked to destabilising warfarin therapy [194], although no interaction was found in a randomised, double-blind trial [195].

Patient Age, Height and Weight

Longitudinal studies to establish how increasing age changes warfarin dose requirement have been performed [196], and it is estimated that warfarin requirement falls by ~20% over a period of 15 years. This decrease in requirement is likely to be a function of a decrease in liver size, and diminished enzyme activity or clotting activity over time [196]. Many studies have shown weight to be an important determinant of warfarin dose requirement. When combined age, height and weight account for approximately 10 – 20% of a patient's warfarin response [197].

Liver Function

Liver dysfunction increases a patient's sensitivity to warfarin through impaired coagulation factor synthesis e.g. the production of proteins that have not been fully γ-carboxylated. Hepatic cirrhosis, a two-fold elevation of liver aspartate aminotransferase (AST), alanine transaminase ALT or an albumin < 3.6 g/L are all indications that special care should be taken during initial anticoagulation.

Kidney Function

Patients with chronic kidney disease and end stage renal disease should be initiated on lower doses of warfarin and monitored closely. These patients are more difficult to control and are at greater risk of haemorrhagic complications [198].

Warfarin Resistance

In a survey of 820 stably anticoagulated patients within an INR range of 2–4, the median daily warfarin dose was 4 mg (range 1–32 mg) and 1% of individuals required a warfarin dose of >20 mg day [168]. We define warfarin resistance as a prolonged warfarin requirement of >20 mg day to achieve therapeutic anticoagulation or failure to achieve therapeutic anticoagulation with this dose [199]. Warfarin-resistant individuals usually present at the start of oral anticoagulation with failure of conventional warfarin-loading regimens to achieve a therapeutic INR. Although, a small proportion of individuals may go on to require increasing doses of warfarin to remain in a therapeutic INR range despite an initial low dose requirement.

Causes of Resistance

Patients with apparent warfarin resistance should be evaluated for compliance, dietary habits and the influence of polypharmacy where applicable. In our experience, non- and intermittent compliance are the most common source of anticoagulation failure.

Non compliance can be detected through the failure to detect circulatory warfarin in a warfarinised patient. Erratic compliance can be more difficult to demonstrate as circulatory levels of warfarin are detected prior to the catabolism of fully functional vitamin K-dependent clotting factors and any resultant increase in the INR. In this situation repeat measurement of the serum warfarin concentration can prove informative since wide variation strongly hints at intermittent compliance.

Genuine warfarin resistance can be subdivided into two broad categories based on whether warfarin resistance arises from abnormal warfarin pharmacokinetics (increased metabolic clearance or decreased absorption of warfarin) or abnormal pharmacodynamics (decreased anticoagulant response). When warfarin is administered to an individual with pharmacokinetic resistance, serum levels decline with an unusually rapid half-life. This most commonly arises through enhanced warfarin metabolism induced through the co-prescription of drugs that increase the activity of the liver cytochrome P450 enzymes. Examples of pharmaceuticals associated with pharmacokinetic warfarin resistance include barbiturates, carbamazepine, griseofulvin and rifampicin [200].

Reduced warfarin absorption is also a form of pharmacokinetic resistance, but since warfarin is absorbed by passive diffusion, malabsorption is extremely uncommon, even in individuals with significant small bowel disease [201]. Warfarin absorption may be diminished when co-prescribed with cholestyramine (cholestyramine binds warfarin within the gut leading to enhanced elimination) [202].

Heritable pharmacokinetic warfarin resistance has been described, most likely due to changes in the genes encoding components of the cytochrome P450 enzyme system [203]. At this time, the large number (>57) of genes responsible for coding the various cytochrome P450 enzymes, plus multiple pseudo-genes, make the investigation of these patients exceedingly time consuming. Table 15 below summarises pharmacokinetic determinants of warfarin resistance.

Table 15. Summary of pharmacokinetic determinants of warfarin resistance

Variable factors (approximate influence on dose requirement)	
Poly pharmacy	many interactions (+ pharmacodynamic)
Co morbidity	renal insufficiency
Fixed factors	
P450 variants (~15%)	
Absorption	
Poor absorption	extremely rare (passive process in stomach and proximal small intestine)

Pharmacodynamic warfarin resistance is indicated when an elevated circulatory warfarin concentration beyond that of the upper limit of the therapeutic range is achieved through high daily doses of warfarin, yet the INR remains consistently sub-therapeutic. It is useful to further sub-classify pharmacodynamic warfarin resistance into pseudo (potentially reversible) and hereditary forms. Pseudo resistance can be induced though the habitual consumption of diets exceptionally rich in vitamin K_1 [204]. The co-prescription of oestrogens can also lead to a form of pseudo pharmacodynamic warfarin resistance through increased vitamin K dependent clotting factor synthesis. Table 16 below summarises pharmacodynamic determinants of warfarin resistance.

Table 16. Summary of pharmacodynamic determinants of warfarin resistance

Variable factors (approximate influence on dose requirement)	
Age (~5%)	warfarin dose response increases with age ~20 % or 15 yr. ? function of decrease in liver size with age ? change in enzyme activity ? clotting factor activity
Liver function	dysfunction leads to increase in response
Height and Weight (~10%)	
Poly pharmacy	many interactions (+ pharmacokinetic)
Co morbidity	e.g. hypertension cerebrovascular disease ischemic stroke serious heart disease malignancy
Vitamin K status	
Fixed factors	
VKORC1 haplotype (up to 40%)	

Once potential sources of pseudo warfarin resistance have been explored and discounted, analysis of the VKORC1 gene should be performed. It is thought that VKORC1 is expressed on the endoplasmic reticulum although there is debate regarding the topology. An early module suggested three trans-membrane domains (TM 1–3), a cytoplasmic loop (CL; residues 31– 100) between TM1 and TM2 and a small luminal loop (residues 121–127) between TM2 and TM3 [205] (although more recent, and yet to be published evidence indicates that four transmembrane domains are likely to exist). The likely redox centre responsible for catalysing the salvaging of K_1O are the cysteine residues located at 132 and 135 within TM3, with an adjacent TYA motif at residues 138–140 conferring a warfarin binding capability [166]. Substitutions within TM3 confer a severe form of pharmacodynamic warfarin resistance possibly as a consequence steric hindrance to warfarin binding [199].

Several nucleotide substitutions have also been identified within the CL of individuals demonstrating pharmacodynamic warfarin resistance [199]. VKORC1 CL contains conserved cysteine residues at 44 and 51 [165]. It has been proposed that the VKORC1 protein possesses an accessory binding site for the 3-substituent of 4-hydroxycoumarins within the CL leading to warfarin resistance [199].

The Laboratory Investigation of Patients with Apparent Warfarin Resistance

The investigation of patients with apparent warfarin resistance can be assessed by performing studies in which the patient is given a supervised oral dose of warfarin. A series of blood samples should then be collected to determine bioavailability, the serum half-life of warfarin and the pharmacodynamic response as evaluated by conventional INR measurements at appropriate times (i.e. baseline, 24, 48 and 72 hours) by the hospital in which the patient is being treated. The warfarin dose used for the study should be equivalent to the current prescribed dose. In our experience up to 0.5 mg/kg is typical. In exceptionally rare cases e.g. if warfarin malabsorption is indicated by the initial oral study, an intravenous dosing study may also be necessary to elucidate the cause of resistance. If both studies need to be conducted a wash-out period of at least two weeks is required between each study. If clinically acceptable, regular warfarin therapy should not be restarted until the end of the 72 hour study period. More frequent sampling is required in the eight-to-12-hour period after administration to measure the peak serum concentration and assess absorption while daily measurements thereafter are sufficient to measure the half-life of clearance of warfarin.

Protocol for the Laboratory Investigation of Apparent Warfarin Resistance

Warfarin Administration:- For the oral study, a single dose of sodium warfarin should be administered in the same tablet form as being prescribed. The tablets should be taken orally in the morning on an empty stomach and swallowed whole with a cup (~100 mL) of water. No food should be taken for at least 2 hours after giving the warfarin. For the intravenous study the same dose of sodium warfarin should be dissolved in sterile water (to be prepared by the local Pharmacy Department). Before starting each study the usual warfarin dose should be withdrawn for not less than 36 hours, and if necessary heparin therapy instituted. Patients with warfarin resistance are often on heparin and this may be continued during the studies.

Blood Samples and Analytical Measurements

- *All time points:*-Serum warfarin:- Blood collected into plain tube and serum separated [206].
- *Baseline, 24, 48, 72 hours:*- Serum vitamin K_1 and vitamin K_1 epoxide:- Blood collected into plain tube and serum separated [207,208] .
- *Baseline, 24, 48, 72 hours*:-Important: Separate in house INR measurements should be performed (citrated blood) to guard against over anticoagulation.

For warfarin and vitamin K assays a single tube of serum may be provided for each time point. Volumes as indicated below. After separation of serum (avoid excessive exposure to light to prevent degradation of vitamin K), store at -20° C or below prior to analysis. Blood sample timings are shown below.

Oral Dosing Study:-Blood sample timings, sample types and volume

0 (baseline)	**3.0 mL** serum + citrate for **INR**
2 hours	1.0 mL serum
4 hours	1.0 mL serum
6 hours	1.0 mLserum
24 hours	**3.0 mL** serum + citrate for **INR**
48 hours	**3.0 mL** serum + citrate for **INR**
72 hours	**3.0 mL** serum + citrate for **INR**

Intravenous Dosing Study:-Blood sample timings, sample types and volumes.

0 (baseline)	**3.0 mL** serum + citrate for **INR**
10 minutes	1.0 mL serum
20 minutes	1.0 mL serum
30 minutes	1.0 mL serum
1 hour	1.0 mL serum
1.5 hours	1.0 mL serum
2 hours	1.0 mL serum
3 hours	1.0 mL serum
4 hours	1.0 mL serum

6 hours	1.0 mL serum
8 to 12 hours	1.0 mL serum
24 hours	**3.0 mL** serum + citrate for **INR**
48 hours	**3.0 mL** serum + citrate for **INR**
72 hours	**3.0 mL** serum + citrate for **INR**

Pharmacology of Warfarin

Warfarin absorption occurs passively in the upper gastrointestinal tract and is detectable in the circulation within one hour of ingestion. Bioavailability is close to 100% with circulatory concentrations of warfarin reaching a maximum two to nine hours after ingestion, where it is highly bound (>97%) to proteins (predominantly to albumin) and shows a clearance half-life ranging from 15 to 58 hours between individuals [209]. In stably anticoagulated patients with an INR in the range 2–4, the serum warfarin concentration reference range is 0.7–2.3 mg/L [168]. In patients on a constant warfarin dose who are fully compliant with treatment, little daily variation in serum warfarin concentration is expected.

Patient Management in Warfarin Resistance

The mechanism of warfarin resistance should be investigated in all patients that encounter sustained difficultly in achieving therapeutic anticoagulation. Once identified reversible causes of warfarin resistance should be corrected where possible. With close monitoring heritable resistance to warfarin at conventional doses can be successfully managed with daily doses in the range 50–100 mg, without adverse events. In our experience individuals who are resistant to warfarin rarely show a more favourable response to other coumarin anticoagulants. Monitored dose escalation with warfarin is preferable to changing to unfamiliar alternative coumarin anticoagulants (especially phenindione, because of its greater toxicity).

CONCLUSION

In experienced hands, warfarin can provide safe and effective anticoagulant treatment for the majority of patients suffering from a wide range of conditions. Despite its limitations the INR system has significantly decreased inter-laboratory variability and facilitated adoption of standard therapeutic ranges worldwide. An informed approach to laboratory analysis can significantly enhance and complement the clinical delivery of anti-coagulant care and further reduce adverse events. Even in the setting of expert clinical and laboratory service delivery, there will always be some patients who do experience adverse events and monitoring difficulties, and facilities and expertise must be available to deal with such occurrences. In patients who appear difficult to stabilise, compliance issues and drug and food interactions should be explored before pharmacokinetic and pharmacodynamic issues and hereditary resistance are considered. A variety of clinical management models have been described which can be tailored to local circumstances to maximise clinical efficacy.

APPENDIX 1

DRUGS WHICH INCREASE ANTICOAGULANT EFFECTS OF WARFARIN

Interacting drug	Additional Comment
Alcohol	Fluctuations in INR particularly in heavy drinkers or those with liver disease
Allopurinol	Anticoagulant effects possibly enhanced – monitor closely
Amiodarone	Slow onset – may persist long after amiodarone is stopped. Monitor closely
Amitriptyline	Can cause unpredictable increases or decreases in INR – monitor closely
Aspirin	Avoid aspirin as analgesic, use paracetamol as safer alternative. Low dose aspirin 75-100mg appears not to interact significantly
Azapropazone	Significant – avoid concomitant use
Bezafibrate	Reduce warfarin dose by one third to a half initially and adjust accordingly – monitor closely
Cefaclor	Cefalexin, cefradine and cefuroxime are safer alternatives
Celecoxib	Rare cases of increased INR and bleeding – monitor closely

Drugs which Increase Anticoagulant Effects of Warfarin (Continued)

Interacting drug	Additional Comment
Ciprofibrate	Reduce warfarin dose by one third to a half initially and adjust accordingly – monitor closely
Ciprofloxacin	Rare but unpredictable - monitor
Clarithromycin	Serious interaction but unpredictable and uncommon - use azithromycin as alternative
Clopidogrel	Increased risk of bleeding due to antiplatelet effect. (Manufacturer advises avoid concomitant use)
Dexamethasone	May enhance or reduce warfarin effects - high doses enhance
Dextropropoxyphene	Rare but unpredictable – monitor closely
Diclofenac	Increased bleeding risk with oral diclofenac. Increased risk of haemorrhage with IV diclofenac - avoid concomitant use
Dipyridamole	Increased risk of mild bleeding due to antiplatelet effect
Erythromycin	Serious but unpredictable. Elderly at greatest risk. Monitor closely
Esomeprazole	Anticoagulant effects possibly enhanced – interactions do not appear to be clinically significant. Monitor
Fenofibrate	Reduce warfarin dose by one third to a half initially and adjust accordingly – monitor closely
Fluoxetine	Isolated reports of raised INR and/or haemorrhage - monitor
Fluvastatin	May increase anticoagulant effects - monitor
Ibuprofen	Anticoagulant effects possibly enhanced – monitor closely
Influenza vaccine	Anticoagulant effects possibly enhanced – monitor closely
Itraconazole	Isolated reports but clinically significant – monitor closely
Ketoconazole	Monitor closely – especially in elderly
Lansoprazole	Anticoagulant effects possibly enhanced although interactions do not appear to be clinically significant. Monitor

Interacting drug	Additional Comment
Mefenamic acid	Anticoagulant effects possibly enhanced – monitor closely
Metronidazole	Avoid where possible. Warfarin dose may need to be reduced by up to half. Monitor closely
Miconazole	Avoid – potentially serious interaction. Use nystatin where possible
Mirtazepine	Anticoagulant effect enhanced – monitor and adjust dose
Ofloxacin	Rare but unpredictable - monitor
Omeprazole	Anticoagulant effects possibly enhanced – occasionally clinically significant interactions occur. Monitor
Orlistat	Manufacturer recommends monitoring of warfarin dose/INR
Paracetamol	Intermittent analgesic use unlikely to affect INR (less than 2.5g/week) Prolonged regular use of high doses have been found to increase INR
Penicillin(s)*	See below*
Phenytoin	May reduce or enhance anticoagulant effects – monitor closely
Piroxicam	Monitor and reduce dose if necessary
Prednisolone	May enhance or reduce warfarin effects -high doses enhance
Propafenone	Monitor and reduce dose if necessary
Rosuvastatin	Anticoagulant effect possibly enhanced – monitor closely
Sibutramine	Increased risk of bleeding – monitor closely
Simvastatin	Generally small clinically irrelevant increase in anticoagulant effects. Monitor initially or after increase in simvastatin dose
Tamoxifen	Monitor and reduce warfarin dose as necessary (may require dose reduction of up to half)
Thyroid Hormones	Monitor and adjust warfarin dose as necessary
Venlafaxine	Anticoagulant effects possibly enhanced – monitor closely

DRUGS WHICH REDUCE ANTICOAGULANT EFFECTS OF WARFARIN

Interacting Drug	Additional Comment
Azathioprine	Monitor as warfarin dose may need to be increased
Carbamazepine	Warfarin dose may need to be increased – monitor closely. No known interaction with oxcarbazepine
Dexamethasone	May enhance or reduce warfarin effects -high doses enhance
Oral contraceptives	Generally avoid in thromboembolic disorders
Phenobarbitone	May require 30-60% increase in warfarin dose. Persists for up to 6 weeks on stopping phenobarbitone - monitor
Phenytoin	May reduce or enhance anticoagulant effects – monitor closely
Prednisolone	May enhance or reduce warfarin effects -high doses enhance
Raloxifene	May antagonise warfarin effect - monitor
Rifabutin	Monitor closely. Reduces anticoagulant effects within 5-7days. Warfarin dose may need to be doubled or trebled and reduced on stopping rifabutin
Rifampicin	Monitor closely. Reduces anticoagulant effects within 5-7days. Warfarin dose may need to be doubled or trebled and reduced on stopping rifampicin
Vitamin K	Consider this interaction if patients are warfarin resistant. Vitamin K may be present in enteral feeds, health foods, food supplements, green tea.

PRODUCTS WITH POTENTIAL INTERACTIONS WITH WARFARIN

Product	**Additional Comment**
Alfalfa	Contains large amounts of vitamin K – can reduce the anticoagulant effect of warfarin
Bilberry	May enhance anticoagulant effect – avoid concomitant use
Chamomile	May increase the risk of bleeding
Chondroitin	Chondroitin has anticoagulant activity and should be avoided
Coenzyme Q10	Reduces anticoagulant effect as structurally similar to vitamin K
Cranberry Juice	Possible enhancement of anticoagulant effect of warfarin – avoid concomitant use
Devil's claw	May enhance the antiplatelet effects of warfarin
Dong Quai	Increased risk of bleeding due to inhibition of COX and platelet aggregation. Reports of increases in INR with concurrent use
Evening Primrose Oil	May increase the risk of bruising and bleeding
Fenugreek	May increase the risk of bleeding
Feverfew	May increase bleeding especially in patients already taking certain anti-clotting medications
Flaxseed Oil	May decrease platelet aggregation and increase bleeding
Fish Oils	Fish oils have anti-platelet effects and may increase the risk of bleeding. Monitor closely
Garlic	Increased risk of bleeding due to inhibition of platelet aggregation. Do not take garlic supplements. Regular ingestion of foods containing small amounts of garlic should not pose a problem
Ginger	Large amounts may increase the risk of bleeding – until more is known, monitor INRs closely
Gingko Biloba	Increased risk of bleeding due to inhibition of platelet aggregation and warfarin metabolism

Products with Potential Interactions with Warfarin (Continued)

Product	Additional Comment
Ginseng	Increased risk of bleeding due to inhibition of platelet aggregation
Glucosamine	Recent reports of increased INR in patients who had just started glucosamine. Avoid concomitant use
Grapefruit Juice	May inhibit metabolism and increase warfarin levels. Avoid or use cautiously
Multivitamin supplements	Use cautiously in patients taking warfarin – may contain ingredients that affect warfarin metabolism e.g. ginseng/bilberry/vitamin E
Red Clover	May increase the risk of bleeding
St John's Wort	Reduces anticoagulant effect of warfarin due to increase in metabolism – avoid concomitant use
Vitamin E	Seems to inhibit platelet aggregation and antagonise the effects of clotting factors. Effects appear to be dose-dependent and are probably clinically significant with 400units/day or more

References

[1] Schofield FW. Damaged sweet clover; the cause of a new disease in cattle simulating haemorrhagic septicemia and blackleg. *J. Am. Vet. Med. Assoc.* 1924; 64: 553–556.

[2] Roderick LM. A problem in the coagulation of the blood; "sweet clover disease of the cattle." *Am. J. Physiol.* 1931; 96: 413–416.

[3] Roderick M, Schalk AF. Studies on sweet clover disease. *Agricultural Experiment Station Bulletin* 250 1931, North Dakota Agricultural College, Fargo.

[4] Link KP. The discovery of dicumarol and its sequels. *Circulation* 1959; 19: 97–107.

[5] Griminger P. Vitamin K antagonists: the first 50 years. *J. Nutr.* 1987; 117: 1325-1329.

[6] Allen EV, Barker NW, Waugh JM. A preparation from spoiled sweet clover [3,3′-Methylene-Bis-(4-Hydroxycoumarin)] which prolongs coagulation and prothrombin time of the blood: a clinical study. *JAMA* 1942; 120: 1009-1015.

[7] Holbrook AM, Pereira JA, Labiris R, McDonald H, Douketis JD, Crowther M, Wells PS. Systematic overview of warfarin and its drug and food interactions. *Arch. Intern. Med.* 2005; 165: 1095–1106.

[8] Bell RG, Matschiner JT. Warfarin and the inhibition of vitamin K activity by an oxide metabolite. *Nature* 1972; 237: 32-33.

[9] Whitlon DS, Sadowski JA, Suttie JW. Mechanism of coumarin action: Significance of vitamin K epoxide reductase inhibition. *Biochemistry* 1978; 17: 1371-1377.

[10] Furie B, Bouchard BA, Furie BC. Vitamin K-dependent biosynthesis of γ-carboxyglutamic acid. *Blood* 1999; 93: 1798-1808.

[11] Moore GW. Normal haemostasis. In: Moore GW, Knight G, Blann AD. *Fundamentals of Biomedical Science. Haematology*. Oxford University Press, UK. 2010.

[12] Leytus SP, Foster DC, Kurachi K, Davie EW. Gene for human factor X: a blood coagulation factor whose gene organization is essentially identical with that of factor IX and protein C. *Biochemistry* 1986; 25: 5098-5102.

[13] Suttie JW. The biochemical basis of warfarin therapy. *Adv. Exp. Med. Biol.* 1987; 214: 3–16.

[14] Poller L. International normalised ratios (INR): the first 20 years. *J. Thromb. Haemost* 2004; 2: 849-860.

[15] Quick AJ. The prothrombin time in haemophilia and in obstructive jaundice. *J. Biol. Chem.* 1935; 109: 73-74.

[16] Hoffman M. A cell-based model of coagulation and the role of factor VIIa. *Blood Rev.* 2003; 17 Suppl 1: S1-5.

[17] Moore GW, Gurney DA. Bleeding disorders and their laboratory investigation. In: Moore GW, Knight G, Blann AD. Fundamentals of Biomedical Science. *Haematology*. Oxford University Press, UK. 2010.

[18] WHO technical report 'Guidelines for thromboplastins and plasma used to control oral anticoagulant therapy' Series 889, 1999 http://www.who.int/bloodproducts/publications/WHO_TRS_889_A3.pdf.

[19] Tomenson JA, Thomson JM. Standardisation of the prothrombin time. In: Thomson JM. *Blood Coagulation and Haemostasis: A practical guide*. Third edition. Churchill Livingstone, Edinburgh, 1985: 370-409.

[20] Tomenson JA. A statistician's independent evaluation. In: van den Besselaar AMHP, Lewis SM, Gralnick HR, eds. *Thromboplastin Calibration and Oral Anticoagulant Control*. Martinus-Nijhoff, Boston 1984: 87-108.

[21] Kitchen S, Jennings I, Woods TA, Preston FE. Local calibration of international normalised ratio improves between laboratory agreement: results from the UK National External Quality Assessment Scheme. UK NEQAS (Blood Coagulation) Steering Committee. *Thromb. Haemost.* 1999; 81: 60-65.

[22] van den Besselaar AM, Houbouyan LL, Aillaud MF, Denson KW, Johnston M, Kitchen S, Lindahl TL, Marren M, Martinuzzo ME, Droullé C, Tripodi A, Vergnes C. Influence of three types of automated coagulometers on the international sensitivity index (ISI) of rabbit,

human and recombinant human tissue factor preparations. A multicentre study. *Thromb. Haemost.* 1999; 81: 66-70.

[23] Chantarangkul V, Tripodi A, Cesana BM, Mannucci PM. Calibration of local systems with lyophilised calibrant plasmas improves the interlaboratory variability of the INR in the Italian External Quality Assessment Scheme. *Thromb. Haemost* 1999; 82: 1621-1626.

[24] van den Besselaar AM, Barrowcliffe TW, Houbouyan-Réveillard LL, Jespersen J, Johnston M, Poller L, Tripodi A; Subcommittee on Control of Anticoagulation of the Scientific and Standardization Committee of the ISTH. Guidelines on preparation, certification, and use of certified plasmas for ISI calibration and INR determination. *J. Thromb. Haemost.* 2004; 2:1946-1953.

[25] Poller L, Keown M, Shepherd SA, Shiach CR, Tabeart S. The effects of freeze drying and freeze drying additives on the prothrombin time and the international sensitivity index. *J. Clin. Pathol.* 1999; 52: 744-748.

[26] van den Besselaar AM, Houbouyan-Reveillard LL, Aillaud MF, Denson KW, Droullé C, Johnston M, Kitchen S, Lindahl TL, Marren M, Martinuzzo ME, Tripodi A, Vergnes C. Multicentre evaluation of lyophilised and deep-frozen plasmas for assignment of the international normalised ratio. *Thromb. Haemost* .1999; 82: 1451-1455.

[27] Arkin C. Do we need the geometric mean as the mean normal value in INR determination? *J. Thromb. Haemost* 2005; 3 Suppl 1: Abstract P1903.

[28] D'Angelo A, Galli L, Lang H. Comparison of mean normal prothrombin time (PT) with PT of fresh normal pooled plasma or of a lyophilized control plasma (R82A) as denominator to express PT results: collaborative study of the International Federation of Clinical Chemistry. *Clin. Chem.* 1997; 43: 2169-2174.

[29] Moore GW, Henley A, Cotton SS, Tugnait S, Rangarajan S. Clinically significant differences between point-of-care analysers and a standard analyser for monitoring the international normalised ratio: a multi-instrument evaluation in a hospital outpatient setting. *Blood Coagul Fibrinolysis* 2007; 18: 287-292.

[30] Tay MH, Tien SL, Chua TSJ, Sim LL, Koh TH. An evaluation of point-of-care instrument for monitoring anticoagulation level in adult cardiac patients. *Singapore Med. J.* 2002; 43: 557-562.

[31] Vacas M, Lafuente PJ, Unanue I, Iriarte JA. Comparative study of two portable systems for oral anticoagulant monitoring. *Hematol. J.* 2005; 5: 35-38.

[32] Gosselin R, Owings JT, White RH, Hutchinson R, Branch J, Mahackian K, Johnston M, Larkin EC. A comparison of point-of-care instruments designed for monitoring oral anticoagulant anticoagulation with standard laboratory methods. *Thromb. Haemost.* 2000; 83: 698-703.

[33] Poller L, Keown M, Chauhan N, van den Besselaar AMHP, Tripodi A, Shiach C, Jespersen J. Reliability of international normalised ratios from two point of care test systems: comparison with conventional methods. *BMJ* 2003; 327: 30.

[34] Shiach CR, Campbell B, Poller L, Keown M, Chauhan N. Reliability of point-of-care prothrombin time testing in a community clinic: a randomised crossover comparison with hospital laboratory testing. *Br. J. Haematol.* 2002; 119: 370-375.

[35] Lizotte A, Quessy I, Vanier MC, Martineau J, Caron S, Darveau M, Dubé A, Gilbert É, Blais N, Lalonde L. Reliability, validity and ease of use of a portable point-of-care coagulation device in a pharmacist-managed anticoagulation clinic. *J. Thromb. Thrombolysis* 2002; 14: 247-254.

[36] Zweig SE. Dry reagent prothrombin time and other haemostasis methods. In: Kost GJ (ed) *Principles and practice of point-of-care testing*. Lippincott, Williams and Wilkins, Philadelphia, USA. 2002: 57-66.

[37] Fitzmaurice DA, Gardiner C, Kitchen S, Mackie I, Murray ET, Machin SJ; British Society of Haematology Taskforce for Haemostasis and Thrombosis. An evidence-based review and guidelines for patient self-testing and management of oral anticoagulation. *Br. J. Haematol.* 2005; 131:156-165.

[38] Connock M, Stevens C, Fry-Smith A, Jowett S, Fitzmaurice D, Moore D, Song F. Clinical effectiveness and cost-effectiveness of different models of managing long-term oral anticoagulation therapy: a systematic review and economic modelling. *Health Technol. Assess* 2007; 11: iii-iv, ix-66.

[39] Gardiner C, Longair I, Pescott MA, Erwin H, Hills J, Machin SJ, Cohen H. Self-monitoring of oral anticoagulation: does it work outside trial conditions? *J. Clin. Pathol.* 2009; 62: 168-171.

[40] Kitchen DP, Kitchen S, Jennings I, Woods T, Walker I. Quality assessment in point-of-care coagulation testing. *Semin .Thromb Haemost* 2008; 34: 647-653.

[41] Horsti J. Agreement of Owren and Quick prothrombin times: effects of citrate and calcium concentrations and international sensitivity index correction. *Clin. Chem.* 2001; 47: 940-944.

[42] Bridgen ML, Graydon C, McLeod B, Lesperance M. Prothrombin time determination. The lack of need for a discard tube and 24-hour stability. *Am. J. Clin. Pathol.* 1997; 108: 422-426.

[43] Moore GW, Rangarajan S, Holland LJ, Henley A, Savidge GF. Low frequency of elevated prothrombin times in patients with lupus anticoagulants when using a recombinant thromboplastin reagent: implications for dosing and monitoring of oral anticoagulant therapy. *Br. J. Biomed. Sci.* 2005; 62: 15-18.

[44] Rosborough TK, Shepherd MF. Unreliability of international normalised ratio for monitoring warfarin therapy in patients with lupus anticoagulant. *Pharmacotherapy* 2004; 24: 838-842.

[45] Ansell J, Hirsh J, Hylek E, Jacobsen A, Crowther M, Palareti G. Pharmacology and management of the vitamin K antagonists: American College of Chest Physicians evidence-based clinical practice guidelines. *Chest* 2008; 133: 160S-198S.

[46] Keeling D, Baglin T, Tait C, Watson H, Perry D, Baglin C, Kitchen S, Makris M. Guidelines on oral anticoagulation with warfarin - fourth edition. *Br. J. Haematol.* 2011; Article first published online: 14 Jun 2011 | DOI: 10.1111/j.1365-2141.2011.08753.x.

[47] Scottish Intercollegiate Guidelines Network (SIGN). Prevention and management of venous thromboembolism. Edinburgh: SIGN; 2010. (SIGN publication no. 122).

[48] Scottish Intercollegiate Guidelines Network (SIGN). Antithrombotic therapy. Edinburgh: SIGN; 1999. (SIGN publication no. 36).

[49] Beinema M, Brouwers JR, Schalekamp T Wilffert B. Pharmacogenetic differences between warfarin, acenocoumarol and phenprocoumon. *Thromb. Haemost* .2008; 100:1052-1057.

[50] Kabat H, Stohlman EF and Smith MI. Hypoprothrombinemia induced by administration of indandione derivatives. *J. Pharmacol. Exp. Ther.* 1944; 80: 160-170.

[51] O'Reilly RA. Vitamin K and the oral anticoagulant drugs. *Annu. Rev. Med.* 1976; 27: 245-261.

[52] Lowenthal J, MacFarlane JA and McDonald KM. The inhibition of the antidotal activity of vitamin K1 against coumarin anticoagulant drugs by its chloro analogue. *Experientia* 1960; 16: 428-429.

[53] Esmon CT and Suttie JW. Vitamin K-dependent carboxylase. Solubilization and properties. *J. Biol. Chem.* 1976; 251: 6238-6243.

[54] Woolly DW. Some biological effects produced by α-tocopherol quinone. *J. Biol. Chem.* 1945; 159: 59-66.

[55] Dowd P and Zheng ZB. On the mechanism of the anticlotting action of vitamin E quinone. *Proc. Natl. Acad. Sci. USA* 1995; 92: 8171-8175.

[56] Marshall FN. 2,3,5,6-tetrachloro-4-pyridinol: a new chemical structure for anticoagulation activity. *Proc. Soc. Exp. Biol. Med.* 1972; 139: 223-22.

[57] Marshall FN. Potency and coagulation factor effects of 2,3,5,6-tetrachloro-4-pyridinol compared to warfarin and its antagonism by vitamin K. *Proc. Soc. Exp. Biol. Med.* 1972; 139: 806-810.

[58] Ren P, Laliberte RE and Bell RG. Effects of warfarin, phenylindanedione, tetrachloropyridinol, and chloro-vitamin K_1 on prothrombin synthesis and vitamin K metabolism in normal and warfarin-resistant rats. *Mol. Pharmacol.* 1974; 10: 373-380.

[59] Bang NU, O'Doherty GOP and Barton RD. Selective suppression of vitamin K-dependent procoagulant synthesis by compounds unrelated to vitamin K. *Clin. Res.* 1975; 23: 521A.

[60] Braidy N, Bui K, Bajorek B. Evaluating the impact of new anticoagulants in the hospital setting. *Pharmacy Practice* 2011; 9:1-10.

[61] Gómez-Moreno G, Aguilar-Salvatierra A, Martín-Piedra MA, Guardia J, Calvo-Guirado JL, Cabrera M, López-Gallardo C, Castillo T. Dabigatran and rivaroxaban, new oral anticoagulants. New approaches in dentistry. *J. Clin. Exp. Dent.* 2010;2:e1-5.

[62] Gage BF, Fihn SD, White RH. Management and dosing of warfarin therapy. *Am. J. Med.* 2000; 109: 481–488.

[63] Levine MN, Raskob G, Landefeld S, Kearon C. Hemorrhagic complications of anticoagulant treatment. *Chest* 2001; 119 (1 Suppl):108S-121S.

[64] Landefeld S, Goldman L. Major bleeding in outpatients treated with warfarin: incidence and prediction by factors known at the start of outpatient therapy. *Am. J. Med.* 1989; 87: 144–152.

[65] Landefeld CS, Beyth RJ. Anticoagulant-related bleeding: clinical epidemiology, prediction, and prevention. *Am. J. Med.* 1993; 95: 315–328.

[66] Landefeld CS, Anderson PA, Goodnough LT, Moir TW, Hom DL, Rosenblatt MW, Goldman L. The bleeding severity index: validation and comparison to other methods for classifying bleeding complications of medical therapy. *J. Clin. Epidemiol.* 1989; 42: 711–718.

[67] Gitter M, Jaeger T, Petterson T, Gersh B, Silverstein M. Bleeding and thromboembolism during anticoagulant therapy: a population-based study in Rochester, Minnesota. *Mayo Clin. Proc.* 1995; 70: 725-733.

[68] van der Meer FJM, Rosendaal FR, Vandenbroucke JP, Briet E. Bleeding complications in oral anticoagulant therapy: an analysis of risk factors. *Arch. Intern. Med.* 1993; 153: 1557-1562.

[69] Cannegieter SC, Rosendaal FR, Wintzen AR, van der Meer FJM, Vandenbroucke JP, Briet E. Optimal oral anticoagulant therapy in patients with mechanical heart valves. *N. Engl. J. Med.* 1995; 333: 11-17.

[70] Levine M, Raskob GE, Landefeld S, Kearon C. Hemorrhagic complications of anticoagulant treatment. *Chest* 1998; 114 Suppl 5: 511S-523S.

[71] Laupacis A, Boysen G, Connolly S, Ezekowitz M, Hart R, James K, Kistler P, Kronmal R, Petersen P, Singer D. Risk factors for stroke and efficacy of antithrombotic therapy in atrial fibrillation. Analysis of pooled data from five randomized controlled trials. *Arch. Intern. Med.* 1994; 154: 1449-1457.

[72] The European Atrial Fibrillation Trial Study Group. Optimal oral anticoagulant therapy in patients with non-rheumatic atrial fibrillation and recent cerebral ischemia. *N. Engl. J. Med.* 1995; 333: 5-10.

[73] The Stroke Prevention in Reversible Ischemia Trial (SPIRIT) Study Group. A randomized trial of anticoagulants versus aspirin after cerebral ischemia of presumed arterial origin. *Ann. Neurol.* 1997; 42: 857-865.

[74] Delaney JA, Opatrny L, Brophy JM, Suissa S. Drug drug interactions between antithrombotic medications and the risk of gastrointestinal bleeding. *CMAJ* 2007; 177: 347–351.

[75] Landefeld S, Beyth RJ. Anticoagulant-related bleeding: clinical epidemiology, prediction and prevention. *Am. J. Med.* 1993; 95: 315-328.

[76] Campbell P, Roberts G, Eaton V, Coghlan D, Gallus A. Managing warfarin therapy in the community. *Aust. Prescr* 2001; 24: 86-89.

[77] Van der Meer FJM, Rosendaal FR, Vandenbroucke JP, Briet E. Bleeding complications in oral anticoagulant therapy: an analysis of risk factors. *Arch. Intern. Med.* 1993; 153: 1557-1562.

[78] Froom P, Miron E, Barak M. Oral anticoagulants in the elderly. *Br. J. Haematol.* 2003; 120: 262-268.

[79] Palareti G, Leali N, Coccheri S, Poggi M, Manotti C, D'Angelo A, Pengo V, Erba N, Moia M, Ciavarella N, Devoto G, Berrettini M, Musolesi S. Bleeding complications of oral anticoagulant treatment: an inception-cohort, prospective collaborative study (ISCOAT). *Lancet* 1996; 348: 423-428.

[80] Borosak M, Choo S, Street A. Warfarin: balancing the benefits and harms. *Aust. Prescr*. 2004;27:88-92.

[81] Lankiewicz MW, Hays J, Friedman KD, Tinkoff G, Blatt PM. Urgent reversal of warfarin with prothrombin complex concentrate. *J. Thromb. Haemost* 2006; 4: 967–970.

[82] Chan YC, Valenti D, Mansfield AO, Stansby G. Warfarin induced skin necrosis. *Br. J. Surg*. 2000; 87: 266–272.

[83] Marlar RA, Neumann A. Neonatal purpura fulminans due to homozygous protein C or protein S deficiencies. *Semin. Thromb. Hemost* 1990; 16: 299-309.

[84] Gage BF, Birman-Deych E, Radford MJ, Nilasena DS, Binder EF. Risk of osteoporotic fracture in elderly patients taking warfarin: results from the National Registry of Atrial Fibrillation 2. *Arch. Intern. Med.* 2006; 166: 241–246.

[85] Koos R, Krueger T, Westenfeld R, Kühl HP, Brandenburg V, Mahnken AH, Stanzel S, Vermeer C, Cranenburg EC, Floege J, Kelm M, Schurgers LJ. Relation of circulating Matrix Gla-Protein and anticoagulation status in patients with aortic valve calcification. *Thromb. Haemost.* 2009; 101: 706-713.

[86] Hyman BT, Landas SK, Ashman RF, Schelper RL, Robinson RA. Warfarin-related purple toes syndrome and cholesterol microe mbolisation. *Am. J. Med.* 1987; 82: 1233–1237.

[87] Talmadge DB, Spyropoulos AC. Purple toes syndrome associated with warfarin therapy in a patient with antiphospholipid syndrome. *Pharmacotherapy* 2003; 23: 674–677.

[88] Zaman S, Mallya J, Thomas M. A man with purple toes. *Postgraduate Medical Journal* 1998;74:51–55.

[89] Holbrook AM, Pereira JA, Labiris R, McDoanld H, Douketis JD, Crowther M, Wells PS. Systematic overview of warfarin and its drug and food interactions. *Arch. Intern. Med.* 2005; 165: 1095-1106.

[90] Raebel MA, Witt DM, Carroll NM, Magid DJ. Warfarin monitoring in ambulatory older individuals receiving antimicrobial therapy. *Pharmacotherapy* 2005; 25: 1055-1061.

[91] Juurlink DN. Drug interactions with warfarin: what clinicians need to know. *CMAJ* 2007; 177: 369–371

[92] Buckley NA, Dawson AH.: Drug interactions with warfarin. *Med. J. Aust* 1992; 157: 479-483.

[93] Weathermon R, Crabb DW. Alcohol and medication interactions. *Alcohol Research and Health* 1999; 23: 40-51.

[94] Havrda DE, Mai T, Chonlahan J. Enhanced antithrombotic effect of warfarin associated with low-dose alcohol consumption. *Pharmacotherapy* 2005; 25: 303-307.

[95] Ruf JC. Alcohol, wine and platelet function. *Biol. Res.* 2004; 37: 209-215.

[96] Renaud SC, Ruf JC. Effects of alcohol on platelet functions. *Clin. Chim. Acta* 1996; 246: 77-89.

[97] Stephens MA, Self TH, Lancaster D, Nash T. Hypothyroidism: effect on warfarin anticoagulation. *South Med. J.* 1989; 82: 1585–1586.

[98] Chute JP, Ryan CP, Sladek G, Shakir KM. Exacerbation of warfarin-induced anticoagulation by hyperthyroidism. *Endocr .Pract.* 1997; 3: 77–79.

[99] Demirkan K, Stephens MA, Newman KP, Self TH. Response to warfarin and other oral anticoagulants: effects of disease states. *South Med. J.* 2000; 93: 448-454.

[100] Lininger SW Gaby AR, Austin S, Batz F, Yarnell E, Brown DJ and Constantine G. *A-Z guide to drug-herb-vitamin interactions.* Prima publishing. Roseville California USA. 1999.

[101] Buckley MS, Goff AD, Knapp WE. Fish Oil interaction with warfarin. *Ann. Pharmacother*. 2004; 38: 50-53.

[102] Dr Jo Barnes BPharm MRPharmS; Working Group on Complementary Medicine (September 2002). "Herb-medicine interactions: St John's Wort (*Hypericum perforatum*) Useful information for pharmacist" (PDF). 1 Lambeth High Street, London SE1 7JN: Royal Pharmaceutical Society of Great Britain. p. 5. http://www.rpsgb.org.uk/pdfs/ scifactsheetstjwort.pdf.

[103] Suvarna R, Pirmohamed M, Henderson L Possible interaction between warfarin and cranberry juice. *BMJ* 2003; 327: 1454.

[104] Aston JL, Lodolce AE, Shapiro NL. Interaction between warfarin and cranberry juice. *Pharmacotherapy* 2006; 9: 1314–1319.

[105] Nutescu EA, Shapiro NL, Ibrahim S, West P. Warfarin and its interactions with foods, herbs and other dietary supplements. *Expert Opin Drug Saf* 2006; 5: 433-451).

[106] Greer IA. The special case of venous thromboembolism in pregnancy. *Haemostasis* 1998; 28 Suppl 3: 22-34.

[107] Ginsberg J, Barron W. Pregnancy and prosthetic heart valves. *Lancet* 1994; 344: 1170-1172.

[108] Schardein JL, Macina OT. *Warfarin. Human Developmental Toxicants*. CRC Taylor and Francis. (2007) Boca Raton, Florida, USA.

[109] Loftus, Christopher M. (1995). "Fetal toxicity of common neurosurgical drugs". *Neurosurgical Aspects of Pregnancy*. Park Ridge, Ill: American Association of Neurological Surgeons.

[110] Hou J. Fetal Warfarin Syndrome. *Chang Gung Med. J*. 2004; 9: 691-695.

[111] Iturbe-Alessio I, del Carmen Fonseca M, Mutchinik O, Santos Ma, Zajarias A, Salazar El. Risks of anticoagulant therapy in pregnant women with artificial heart valves. *N. Engl. J. Med*. 1986; 315: 1390-1393.

[112] Orme ML, Lewis PJ, de Swiet M, Serlin MJ, Sibeon R, Baty JD, Breckenridge AM. May mothers given warfarin breast-feed their infants? *BMJ* 1977; 1: 1564-1565.

[113] Kovacs MJ, Rodger M, Anderson DR, Morrow B, Kells G, Kovacs J, Boyle E, Wells PS. Comparison of 10-mg and 5-mg warfarin initiation nomograms together with low-molecular-weight heparin for outpatient treatment of acute venous thromboembolism. A randomized, double-blind, controlled trial. *Ann. Intern. Med*. 2003; 138: 714–719.

[114] Fennerty A, Campbell IA, Routledge PA. Anticoagulants in venous thromboembolism. *BMJ* 1988; 297: 1285–1288.

[115] Tait RC, Sefcick A. A warfarin induction regimen for out-patient anticoagulation in patients with atrial fibrillation. *Br. J. Haematol.* 1998; 101: 450–454.

[116] Lenzini P, Grice G, Milligan P, Gatchel S, Deych E, Eby C, Burnett R, Clohisy J, Barrack R, Gage B. Optimal initial dose adjustment of warfarin in orthopedic patients. *Ann. Pharmacother.* 2007; 41: 1798-1804.

[117] Hirsh J, Fuster V, Ansell J, Halperin JL. American Heart Association /American College of Cardiology Foundation Guide to Warfarin Therapy. *Circulation* 2003; 107: 1692-1711

[118] Walker ID, Machin S, Baglin TP, Barrowcliffe TW, Colvin BT, Greaves M, Ludlam CA, Mackie IJ, Preston FE, Rose PE. Guidelines on oral anticoagulation: third edition. *Br. J. Haematol.* 1998; 101: 374-387.

[119] Kearon C, Hirsh J. Management of anticoagulation before and after elective surgery. *N. Engl. J. Med.* 1997; 336: 1506-1511.

[120] Baughman KL. Valvular heart disease. In: Colman RW, Marder VJ, Clowes AW, George JN, Goldhaber SZ (Eds). Hemostasis and Thrombosis: Basic principles and clinical practice. 5th edition. 2006 Lippincott Williams and Wilkins, Philadelphia, PA USA.

[121] Hyers TM, Agnelli G, Hull RD, Weg JG, Morris TA, Samama M, Tapson V. Antithrombotic therapy for venous thromboembolic disease. *Chest* 1998; 114 Suppl 5: 561S-578S.

[122] Kuijer, PMM, Prins, MH, Buller, HR Low-molecular-weight heparins: treatment of venous thromboembolism. In: Sasahara AA, Loscalzo J (eds). *Advances in therapeutic agents in thrombosis and thrombolysis.* 1997,129-147 Marcel Dekker. New York, NY.

[123] Simonneau, G, Sors, H, Charbonnier, B, Page Y, Laaban JP, Azarian R, Laurent M, Hirsch JL, Ferrari E, Bosson JL, Mottier D, Beau B. A comparison of low-molecular-weight heparin with unfractionated heparin for acute pulmonary embolism. The THESEE Study Group. *N. Engl. J. Med.* 1997; 337: 663-669.

[124] Levine, M, Gent, M, Hirsh, J, Leclerc J, Anderson D, Weitz J, Ginsberg J, Turpie AG, Demers C, Kovacs M. A comparison of low molecular weight heparin administered primarily at home with UFH administered in the hospital for proximal deep vein thrombosis. *N. Engl. J. Med.* 1996; 334: 677-681.

[125] Segal JB, Streiff MB, Hofmann LV, Hoffman LV, Thornton K, Bass EB.Management of venous thromboembolism: a systematic review for a practice guideline. *Ann. Intern. Med.* 2007; 146: 211-222.

[126] Optimum duration of anticoagulation for deep-vein thrombosis and pulmonary embolism. Research Committee of the British Thoracic Society. *Lancet* 1992; 340: 873-876.

[127] Schulman S, Rhedin AS, Lindmarker P, Carlsson A, Lärfars G, Nicol P, Loogna E, Svensson E, Ljungberg B, Walter H. A Comparison of six weeks with six months of oral anticoagulation therapy after a first episode of venous thromboembolism. Duration of anticoagulation Trial Study Group. *N. Engl. J. Med.* 1995; 332: 1661-1665.

[128] Schulman S, Granqvist S, Holmstrom M, Carlsson A, Lindmarker P, Nicol P, Eklund SG, Nordlander S, Lärfars G, Leijd B, Linder O, Loogna E. The duration of oral anticoagulant therapy after a second episode of venous thromboembolism. *N. Engl. J. Med.* 1997; 336: 393-398.

[129] Van den Belt AGM, Sanson B-J, Simioni P, Prandoni P, Büller HR, Girolami A, Prins MH. Recurrence of venous thromboembolism in patients with familial thrombophilia. *Arch. Intern. Med.* 1997; 157: 2227-2232.

[130] Lagerstedt CI, Olsson C-G, Fagher BO, Oqvist BW, Albrechtsson U. Need for long-term anticoagulant treatment in symptomatic calf-vein thrombosis. *Lancet* 1985; 326: 515-518.

[131] Wells PS, Anderson DR, Bormanis J, Guy F, Mitchell M, Gray L, Clement C, Robinson KS, Lewandowski B. Value of assessment of pretest probability of deep-vein thrombosis in clinical management. *Lancet* 1997; 350: 1795-1798.

[132] Wells PS, Anderson DR, Rodger M, Forgie M, Kearon C, Dreyer J, Kovacs G, Mitchell M, Lewandowski B, Kovacs MJ. Evaluation of D-dimer in the diagnosis of suspected deep-vein thrombosis. *N. Engl. J. Med.* 2003; 349: 1227-1235.

[133] Wells P, Anderson D, Rodger M, Ginsberg J, Kearon C, Gent M, Turpie A, Bormanis J, Weitz J, Chamberlain M, Bowie D, Barnes D, Hirsh J. Derivation of a simple clinical model to categorize patients probability of pulmonary embolism: increasing the models utility with the SimpliRED D-dimer. *Thromb. Haemost.* 2000; 83: 416–420.

[134] Subramaniam RM, Chou T, Heath R, Allen R. Importance of pretest probability score and D-dimer assay before sonography for lower limb deep venous thrombosis. *Am. J. Roentgenol.* 2006; 186: 206-212.

[135] van der Velde EF, Toll DB, Ten Cate-Hoek AJ, Oudega R, Stoffers HE, Bossuyt PM, Büller HR, Prins MH, Hoes AW, Moons KG, van Weert HC. Comparing the diagnostic performance of 2 clinical decision rules to rule out deep vein thrombosis in primary care patients. *Ann. Fam. Med.* 2011;9:31-36.

[136] Scarvelis D, Wells P. Diagnosis and treatment of deep-vein thrombosis. *CMAJ* 2006; 175: 1087–1092.

[137] Ost D, Tepper J, Mihara H, Lander O, Heinzer R, Fein A. Duration of anticoagulation following venous thromboembolism: a meta-analysis. *JAMA* 2005; 294: 706-715

[138] Kearon C, Gent M, Hirsh J, Weitz J, Kovacs MJ, Anderson DR, Turpie AG, Green D, Ginsberg JS, Wells P, MacKinnon B, Julian JA. A comparison of three months of anticoagulation with extended anti coagulation for a first episode of idiopathic venous thromboembolism. *N. Engl. J. Med.* 1999; 340: 901-907.

[139] Singer DE. Overview of the randomized trials to prevent stroke in atrial fibrillation. *Ann. Epidemiol.* 1993; 3: 563-567.

[140] Laupacis A, Albers GW, Dalen JE, Dalen J, Dunn MI, Jacobson AK, Singer DE. Antithrombotic therapy in atrial fibrillation. *Chest* 1998; 114 *Suppl.* 5: 579S-589S.

[141] Go AS, Hylek EM, Phillips K, Chang Y, Henault LE, Selby JV, Singer DE. Prevelence of diagnosed atrial fibrillation in adults: national implications for rhythm management and stroke prevention: the AnTicoagulation and Risk Factors in Atrial Fibrilation (ATRIA) Study. *JAMA* 2001; 285: 2370-2375.

[142] Wolf PA, Abbott RD, Kannel WB. Atrial fibrilation as an independent risk factor for stroke: the Framingham Study. *Stroke* 1991; 22: 983-988.

[143] Frost L, Engholm G, Johnsen S, Møller H, Husted S. Incident stroke after discharge from hospital with a diagnosis of atrial fibrillation. *Am. J. Med.* 2000; 108: 36-40.

[144] Hylek EM, Skates SJ, Sheehan MA, Singer DE. An analysis of the lowest effective intensity of prophylactic anticoagulation for patients with non-rheumatic atrial fibrillation. *N. Engl. J. Med.* 1996; 335: 540-546.

[145] Gage BF, Waterman AD, Shannon W, Boechler M, Rich MW, Radford MJ. Validation of clinical classification schemes for predicting stroke. Results from the National Registry of Atrial Fibrillation. *JAMA* 2001; 285: 2864-2870.

[146] European Heart Rhythm Association; European Association for Cardio-Thoracic Surgery, Camm AJ, Kirchhof P, Lip GY, Schotten U, Savelieva I, Ernst S, Van Gelder IC, Al-Attar N, Hindricks G, Prendergast B, Heidbuchel H, Alfieri O, Angelini A, Atar D, Colonna P, De Caterina R, De Sutter J, Goette A, Gorenek B, Heldal M, Hohloser SH, Kolh P, Le Heuzey JY, Ponikowski P, Rutten FH. Guidelines for the management of atrial fibrillation: the Task Force for the Management of Atrial Fibrillation of the European Society of Cardiology (ESC). *Eur. Heart J.* 2010; 31: 2369-2429.

[147] Lip GY, Gibbs CR. Anticoagulation for heart failure in sinus rhythm: a Cochrane systematic review. *QJM* 2002; 95: 451-459.

[148] Lip GY, Gibbs CR. Antiplatelet agents versus control or anticoagulation for heart failure in sinus rhythm: a Cochrane systematic review. *QJM* 2002; 95: 461-468.

[149] Stein PD, Alpert JS, Dalen JE, Horstkotte D, Turpie AG. Antithrombotic therapy in patients with mechanical and biological prosthetic heart valves. *Chest* 1998; 114 Suppl 5: 602S-610S.

[150] Cappelleri JC, Fiore LD, Brophy MT, Deykin D, Lau J. Efficacy and safety of combined anticoagulant and antiplatelet therapy versus anticoagulant monotherapy after mechanical heart-valve replacement: a meta-analysis. *Am. Heart J.* 1995; 130: 547-552.

[151] Chiquette E, Amato MG, Bussey HJ. Comparison of an anticoagulation clinic with usual medical care: Anticoagulation control, patient outcomes and health care costs. *Arch. Intern. Med.* 1998; 158: 1641-1647.

[152] Jacobson AK. In: Ansell JE, Oertel LB, Wittowsky AK, (eds). Managing Oral Anticoagulation Therapy. 2nd ed. St Louis, MO: *Facts and Comparisons;* 2003: 45: 1-6.

[153] Ansell JE, Hughes R. Evolving models of warfarin management: Anticoagulation clinics, patient self-monitoring, and patient self-management. *Am. Heart J.* 1996; 132: 1095-1100.

[154] Gardiner C, Williams K, Longair I, Mackie IJ, Machin SJ, Cohen H. A randomised control trial of patient self-management of oral anti coagulation compared with patient self-testing. *Br. J. Haematol.* 2006; 132: 598-603.

[155] Ansell J, Jacobson A, Levy J, Völler H, Hasenkam JM. Guidelines for implementation of patient self-testing and patient self-management of oral anticoagulation. International consensus guidelines prepared by

International Self-Monitoring Association for Oral Anticoagulation. *Int. J. Cardiol.* 2005; 99: 37-45.

[156] Siebenhofer A, Berghold A, Sawicki PT. Systematic review of studies of self-management of oral anticoagulation . *Thromb. Haemost* 2004; 91: 225-232.

[157] Wittkowsky AK, Sekreta CM, Nutescu EA, Ansell JA. Barriers to patient self-testing of prothrombin time. A national survey of anticoagulation practitioners. *Pharmacotherapy*. 2005; 25: 265-269.

[158] Heneghan C, Alonso-Coello P, Garcia-Alamino JM, Perera R, Meats E, Glasziou P. Self-monitoring of oral anticoagulation: a systematic review and meta-analysis. *Lancet,* 2006; 367: 404-411.

[159] Garcia DA, Witt DM, Hylek E, Wittkowsky AK, Nutescu EA, Jacobson A, Moll S, Merli GJ, Crowther M, Earl L, Becker RC, Oertel L, Jaffer A, Ansell JE. Delivery of optimized anticoagulant therapy: consensus statement from the Anticoagulation Forum. *Ann. Pharmacother* 2008; 42: 979-988.

[160] Campbell P, Radensky P, Denham C. Economic analysis of systematic anticoagulation management vs. routine medical care for patients on oral warfarin therapy. *Dis. Manag Clin. Outcome* 2000; 2: 101-108.

[161] Giles TD, Roffidal L. Results of the Prothrombin Office-Testing Benefit Evaluation (PROBE). *CVR&R*. 2002; 23: 27-28,30,32-33.

[162] O'Reilly RA, Aggler PM, Hoag MS, Leong LS, Kropatkin ML. Hereditary transmission of exceptional resistance to coumarin anticoagulant drugs. The first reported kindred. *N Engl. J. Med*. 1964; 15: 809-815.

[163] Bays RP. Unusual sensitivity to warfarin sodium. *J. LA State Med. Soc* 1965; 117: 55-59.

[164] Rettie AE, Jones JP. Clinical and toxicological relevance of CYP2C9: drug-drug interactions and pharmacogenetics. *Annu. Rev. Pharmacol Toxicol.* 2005; 45: 477–494.

[165] Goodstadt L, Ponting CP. Vitamin K epoxide reductase: homology, active site and catalytic mechanism. *Trends Biochem. Sci*. 2004; 29: 289–292.

[166] Rost S, Fregin A, Hunerberg M, Bevans CG, Muller CR, Oldenburg J. Site-directed mutagenesis of coumarin-type anticoagulant-sensitive VKORC1: evidence that highly conserved amino acids define structural requirements for enzymatic activity and inhibition by warfarin. *Thromb Haemost* 2005; 94: 780–786.

[167] Ma Q, Cui K, Xiao F, Lu AY, Yang CS. Identification of a glycinerich sequence as an NAD(P)H-binding site and tyrosine 128 as a dicumarol-binding site in rat liver NAD(P)H: quinone oxidoreductase by site-directed mutagenesis. *J. Biol. Chem.* 1992; 267: 22298–304.

[168] Harrington DJ, Underwood S, Morse C, Shearer MJ, Tuddenham EG, Mumford AD. Pharmacodynamic resistance to warfarin associated with a Val66Met substitution in vitamin K epoxide reductase complex subunit 1. *Thromb Haemost* 2005; 93: 23–26.

[169] D'Ambrosio RL, D'Andrea G, Cappucci F, Chetta M, Di Perna P, Brancaccio V, Grandone E, Margaglione M. Polymorphisms in factor II and factor VII genes modulate oral anticoagulation with warfarin. *Haematologica* 2004; 89: 1510-1516.

[170] Chu K, Wu SM, Stanley T, Stafford DW, High KA. A mutation in the propeptide of Factor IX leads to warfarin sensitivity by a novel mechanism. *J. Clin. Invest* 1996; 98:1619-1625.

[171] Ulrich S, Brand B, Speich R, Oldenburg J, Asmis L. Congenital hypersensitivity to vitamin K antagonists due to FIX propeptide mutation at locus -10: a (not so) rare cause of bleeding under oral anticoagulant therapy in Switzerland. *Swiss Med. Wkly* 2008; 138: 100-107.

[172] Chen LY, Eriksson N, Gwilliam R, Bentley D, Deloukas P, Wadelius M. Gamma-glutamyl carboxylase (GGCX) microsatellite and warfarin dosing. *Blood* 2005; 106: 3673-3674.

[173] Stehle S, Kirchheiner J, Lazar A, Fuhr U. Pharmacogenetics of oral anticoagulants: a basis for dose individualization. *Clin. Pharmacokinet* 2008; 47: 565-594.

[174] Schurgers LJ, Geleijnse JM, Grobbee DE, Pols HAP, Hofman A, Witteman JCM and Vermeer C. Nutritional intake of vitamin K-1 (phylloquinone) and K-2 (menaquinone) in the Netherlands. *J. Nutr. Environm. Med.* 1999; 9: 115-122.

[175] Schurgers LJ and Vermeer C. Determination of phylloquinone and menaquinones in food. Effect of food matrix on circulating vitamin K concentrations. *Haemostasis* 2000; 30: 298-307.

[176] Shearer MJ.Vitamin K metabolism and nutriture. *Blood Rev.* 1992; 6: 92-104.

[177] Suttie JW. The importance of menaquinones in human nutrition. *Annu. Rev. Nutr.* 1995; 15: 399-417.

[178] Booth SL, Price RJ, Weihrauch JL and Ferland G. Vitamin K1 (phylloquinone) content of foods: A provisional table. *J. Food Comp. Anal.* 1993; 6: 109-120.

[179] Bolton-Smith C, Price RG, Fenton ST, Harrington DJ and Shearer MJ. Compilation of a provisional UK database for the phylloquinone (vitamin K1) content of foods. *Br. J. Nutr.* 2000; 83: 389-399.

[180] Shearer MJ, Bach A and Kohlmeier M. Chemistry, nutritional sources, tissue distribution and metabolism of vitamin K with special reference to bone health. *J. Nutr.* 1996; 126 (Suppl 4); 1181S-1186S.

[181] Fenton ST, Price RJ, Bolton-Smith C, Harrington DJ and Shearer MJ. Nutrient sources of phylloquinone (vitamin K1) in Scottish men and women. *Proc. Nutr .Soc.* 1997; 56: 301A.

[182] Tsukamoto Y, Ichise H, Kakuda H and Yamaguchi M. Intake of fermented soybean (natto) increases circulating vitamin K2 (menaquinone-7) and γ-carboxylated osteocalcin concentration in normal individuals. *J. Bone Miner Metab.* 2000; 18: 216-222.

[183] Sobczyńska-Malefora A, Harrington DJ, Lomer MC, Pettitt C, Hamilton S, Rangarajan S, Shearer MJ. Erythrocyte folate and 5-methyltetrahydrofolate levels decline during 6 months of oral anticoagulation with warfarin. *Blood Coagul Fibrinolysis* 2009; 20: 297-302.

[184] Sconce E, Avery P, Wynne H, Kamali F. Vitamin K supplementation can improve stability of anticoagulation for patients with unexplained variability in response to warfarin. *Blood* 2007; 109: 2419–2423.

[185] Rombouts EK, Rosendaal FR, Van Der Meer FJ. Daily vitamin K supplementation improves anticoagulant stability. *J. Thromb. Haemost* 2007; 5: 2043–2048.

[186] Schurgers LJ, Teunissen KJ, Hamulyák K, Knapen MH, Vik H, Vermeer C. Vitamin K-containing dietary supplements: comparison of synthetic vitamin K1 and natto-derived menaquinone-7. *Blood* 2007; 109: 3279-3283.

[187] Conly JM and Stein K. Quantitative and qualitative measurements of K vitamins in human intestinal contents. *Am. J. Gastroenterol.* 1992; 87: 311-316.

[188] Ramotar K, Conly JM, Chubb H and Louie TJ. Production of menaquinones by intestinal anaerobes. *J. Infect Dis*. 1984; 150: 213-218.

[189] Ichihashi T, Takagishi Y, Uchida K and Yamada H. Colonic absorption of menaquinone-4 and menaquinone-9 in rats. *J. Nutr*. 1992; 122: 506-512.

[190] Frick PG, Riedler G and Brögli H. Dose response and minimal daily requirement for vitamin K in man. *J. Appl. Physiol*. 1967; 23: 387-389.

[191] British National Formulary 57. March 2009.

[192] Shearer MJ, Bechtold H, Andrassy K, Koderisch J. McCarthy PT. Trenk D. Jahnchen E. Ritz E. Mechanism of cephalosporin-induced hypoprothrombinemia: relation to cephalosporin side chain, vitamin K metabolism, and vitamin K status. *J. Clin. Pharmacol*. 1988; 28: 88–95.

[193] Thijssen HHW, Soute BA, Vervoort LM and Claessens JG. Paracetamol (acetaminophen) warfarin interaction: NAPQ1, the toxic metabolite of paracetamol, is an inhibitor of enzymes in the vitamin K cycle. *Thromb. Haemost* 2004; 92: 797-802.

[194] Pham DQ, Pham AQ. Interaction potential between cranberry juice and warfarin. *Am. J. Health Syst. Pharm*. 2007; 64: 490-494.

[195] Ansell J, McDonough M, Zhao Y, Harmatz JS, Greenblatt DJ. The absence of an interaction between warfarin and cranberry juice: a randomized, double-blind trial. *J. Clin. Pharmacol*. 2009; 49: 824-830.

[196] Wynne HA, Kamali F, Edwards C, Long A, Kelly P. Effect of ageing upon warfarin dose requirements: a longitudinal study. *Age Ageing* 1996; 25: 429-431.

[197] Jonas DE, McLeod HL. Genetic and clinical factors relating to warfarin dosing. *Trends Pharmacol. Sci*. 2009; 30: 375-386.

[198] Limdi NA, Beasley TM, Baird MF, Goldstein JA, McGwin G, Arnett DK, Acton RT, Allon M. Kidney function influences warfarin responsiveness and hemorrhagic complications. *J. Am. Soc. Nephrol*. 2009; 20: 912-921.

[199] Harrington DJ, Gorska R, Wheeler R, Davidson S, Murden S, Morse C, Shearer MJ, Mumford AD. Pharmacodynamic resistance to warfarin is associated with nucleotide substitutions in VKORC1. *J. Thromb. Haemost*. 2008; 6: 1663-1670.

[200] Holbrook AM, Pereira JA, Labiris R, McDonald H, Douketis JD, Crowther M, Wells PS. Systematic overview of warfarin and its drug and food interactions. *Arch. Intern. Med*. 2005; 165: 1095–1106.

[201] Talstad I, Gamst ON. Warfarin resistance due to malabsorption. *J. Intern. Med.* 1994; 236: 465–467.

[202] Jahnchen E, Meinertz T, Gilfrich HJ, Kersting F, Groth U. Enhanced elimination of warfarin during treatment with cholestyramine. *Br. J. Clin. Pharmacol.* 1978; 5: 437–440.

[203] Ingelman-Sundberg M, Oscarson M, McLellan RA. Polymorphic human cytochrome P450 enzymes: an opportunity for individualized drug treatment. *Trends Pharmacol. Sci.* 1999; 20: 342–349.

[204] Kempin SJ. Warfarin resistance caused by broccoli. *N. Engl. J. Med.* 1983; 08: 1229-1230.

[205] Tie JK, Nicchitta C, von Heijne G, Stafford DW. Membrane topology mapping of vitamin K epoxide reductase by in vitro translation /cotranslocation. *J. Biol. Chem.* 2005; 280: 16410–16416.

[206] Shearer MJ. Assay of coumarin antagonists of vitamin K in blood by high-performance liquid chromatography. *Methods Enzymol* 1986; 123: 223-234.

[207] Davidson KW, Sadowski JA. Determination of vitamin K compounds in plasma or serum by high-performance liquid chromatography using postcolumn chemical reduction and fluorimetric detection. *Methods Enzymol.* 1997; 282: 408-421.

[208] McCarthy PT, Harrington DJ, Shearer MJ. Assay of phylloquinone in plasma by high-performance liquid chromatography with electrochemical detection. *Methods Enzymol.* 1997; 282: 421-433.

[209] O'Reilly RA, Aggeler PM, Leong LS. Studies on the coumarin anticoagulant drugs: the pharmacodynamics of warfarin in man. *J. Clin. Invest* 1963; 42: 1542–1551.

Biographies

Dr Gary W. Moore, Consultant Biomedical Scientist, Centre for Haemostasis and Thrombosis, Diagnostic Haemostasis and Thrombosis Laboratories, GSTS Pathology, Guy's and St. Thomas' NHS Foundation Trust, London, UK.

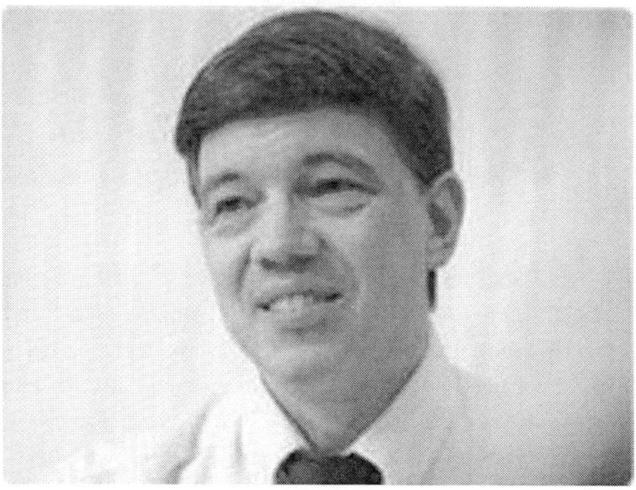

He has been head of the Diagnostic Haemostasis and Thrombosis Laboratories in Guy's and St. Thomas' NHS Foundation Trust since 1997 and maintains a specific interest in lupus anticoagulant detection and screening for hereditary thrombophilias. His publication record has mainly focused on design, modification and interpretation of lupus anticoagulant assays. Gary's other main professional interest involves educational activities whereby he is a visiting specialist lecturer at a number of UK universities and is the Chief Examiner in Haematology for the Institute of Biomedical Science in the UK.

Dr Graeme A. Thomson, Associate Specialist, Centre for Haemostasis and Thrombosis, Guy's and St. Thomas' NHS Foundation Trust, London, UK.

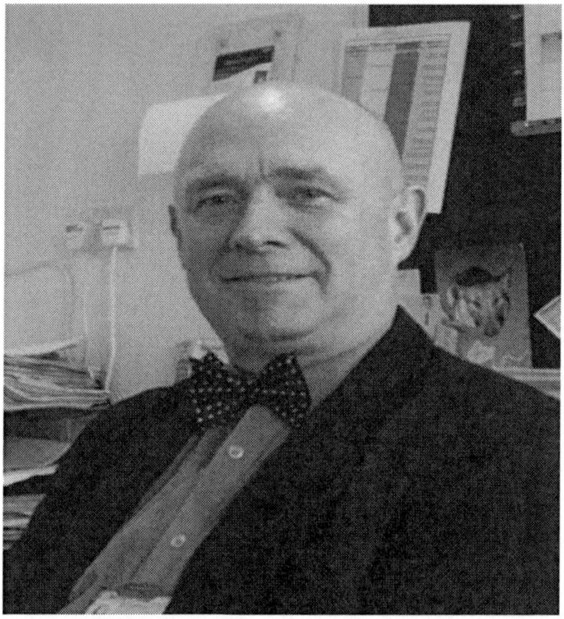

He has been Lead for the anticoagulation service at Guy's and St Thomas' Hospital since 2006 and prior to this was employed at the Chelsea and Westminster Hospital, London where he was extensively involved with the anticoagulation service. His other work within the Centre for Haemostasis and Thrombosis involves both inherited bleeding disorders together with thrombosis and he has a particular interest in the "bridging" of anticoagulation.

Dr Dominic J. Harrington, Consultant Clinical Scientist, Centre for Haemostasis and Thrombosis, Nutristasis Laboratories, GSTS Pathology, Guy's and St. Thomas' NHS Foundation Trust, London, UK and Honorary Senior Lecturer (King's College London).

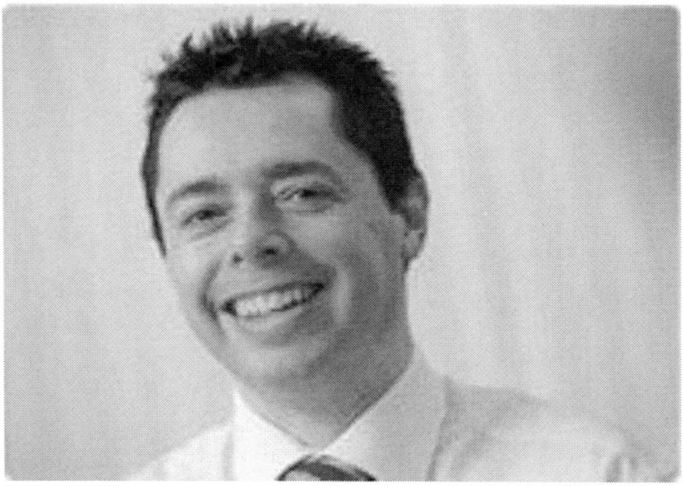

He has a longstanding interest in the use of blood concentrations of vitamins and their respective functional indicators to define status. Dominic established the Nutristasis Unit and has a proven track record in the development and clinical application of novel assays, with special reference to haemostasis and thrombosis. His publication record is predominantly focused on vitamin K and the study of oral anticoagulation resistance. Dominic is the Director of the UK NEQAS vitamin K (KEQAS) quality assurance programme and is a Chartered Quality Professional (Institute of Quality Assurance).

INDEX